I0031939

CLASSIC SERIES

Greatest.

Adventure Stories of
Sherlock Holmes

②

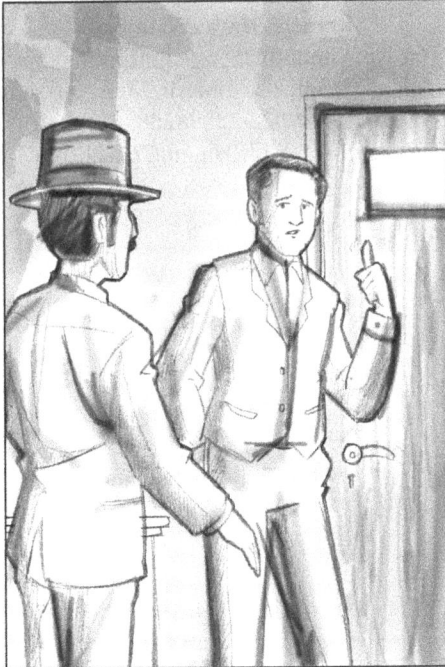

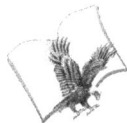

V&S PUBLISHERS

Published by:

V&S PUBLISHERS

F-2/16, Ansari road, Daryaganj, New Delhi-110002
☎ 23240026, 23240027 • *Fax:* 011-23240028
Email: info@vspublishers.com • *Website:* www.vspublishers.com

Regional Office : Hyderabad

5-1-707/1, Brij Bhawan (Beside Central Bank of India Lane)
Bank Street, Koti, Hyderabad - 500 095
☎ 040-24737290
E-mail: vspublishershyd@gmail.com

Branch Office : Mumbai

Flat No. Ground Floor, Sonmegh Building
No. 51, Karel Wadi, Thakurdwar, Mumbai - 400 002
☎ 022-22098268
E-mail: vspublishersmum@gmail.com

Follow us on:

For any assistance sms **VSPUB** to **56161**

All books available at **www.vspublishers.com**

© **Copyright:** *V&S* PUBLISHERS
ISBN 978-93-505710-0-2
Edition 2014

The Copyright of this book, as well as all matter contained herein (including illustrations) rests with the Publishers. No person shall copy the name of the book, its title design, matter and illustrations in any form and in any language, totally or partially or in any distorted form. Anybody doing so shall face legal action and will be responsible for damages.

Printed at : Param Offseters, Okhla, New Delhi-110020

Publisher's Note

It has been our constant endeavour at the **V&S Publishers** to publish all kinds of books ranging from Fiction, Non-fiction, Storybooks, Children Encyclopaedias, to Self-Help, Science Books, Dictionaries, Grammar Books, Self-Development, Management Books, etc.

However, this is for the first time that we are venturing into the vast, rich and fathomless ocean of English Literature and have come up with a set *of ten storybooks called the Greatest Classic Series* authored by some of the greatest and eminent writers of the world. There is a lot to learn from their writing style, selection of plot, development and building of theme and suspense of the story, emphasis and presentation of characters, dialogues, working towards the climax of the story, presenting the climax, and then finally concluding the story.

Each these books are of about 200 pages containing around ten popular stories or more of renowned authors like Oscar Wilde, Ernest William Hornung, Guy de Maupassant, O. Henry, Saki, Washington Irving, Thomas Hardy, Charles Dickens, Jules Verne, Jack London, Mark Twain, Edgar Allen Poe, H.G.Wells, Ambrose Bierce, Amelia Edwards, Edith Wharton, Wilkie Collins and many more. The series is called The Greatest Classic Series as all the names of the books begin with the word, `Greatest' like the Greatest Adventurous Stories, Greatest Detective Stories, Greatest Love Stories, Greatest Ghost Stories, and so on. Besides this, three of the ten books are exclusively on the Adventures of Sherlock Holmes, one of the best detectives the world has ever known written by none other than Sir Arthur Conan Doyle.

Besides the above mentioned characteristics, the books contain an introductory page before each story introducing the author, his brief life history, notable works and literary achievements. Each story has a set of word meanings on each page followed by an exercise meant exclusively aiming the school students to help them grasp the essence of the story easily and quickly.

These books are not only a boon for the school-going students, particularly studying in senior classes from the seventh standard till the twelfth, but are also a treasure trove for all those young and aspiring writers, voracious readers and lovers of English language and literature.

Each of these ten books focus on a theme, such as adventure, love, terror, humour, or supernatural happenings, and are so captivating and real to life that readers may find it difficult to choose from them and so it's better to pick the entire series.

Wishing you all a happy and enjoyable reading…

Contents

Sir Arthur Conan Doyle

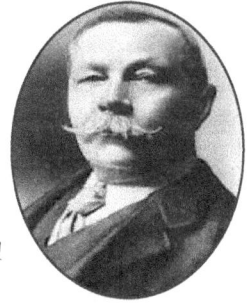

Born on May 22, 1859
Died on July 7, 1930
Notable Works: *Stories of Sherlock Holmes, The Lost World, A Study in Scarlet, etc.*
Honours: Knight Bachelor (1902) and Archie Goodwin Award (2005)

Early Life

Sir Arthur Ignatius Conan Doyle, DL (a Deputy Lieutenant is a military commission in the United Kingdom and one of the several deputies to the Lord Lieutenant of a lieutenancy area) was born on May 22, 1859 at 11 Picardy Place, Edinburgh, Scotland. He was a Scottish physician and writer, most noted for his stories about **the detective, Sherlock Holmes**, generally considered a milestone in the field of crime fiction, and for the **adventures of Professor Challenger**. He was a prolific writer, whose other works include science fiction stories, plays, romances, poetry, non-fiction and historical novels.

His father, Charles Altamont Doyle, was an English of Irish descent, and his mother was an Irish. Although he is now referred to as "Conan Doyle", the origin of this compound surname is uncertain. Supported by wealthy uncles, Conan Doyle was sent to the Roman Catholic Jesuit preparatory school, Hodder Place, Stonyhurst, at the age of nine. He then went on to Stonyhurst College until 1875. From 1875 to 1876, he was educated at the Jesuit school Stella Matutina in Feldkirch, Austria. From 1876 to 1881, he studied medicine at the University of Edinburgh, including a period working in the town of Aston (now a district of Birmingham) and in Sheffield, as well as in Shropshire at Ruyton-XI-Towns. Conan Doyle began writing short stories while studying. His earliest extant fiction, "The Haunted Grange of Goresthorpe", was unsuccessfully submitted to Blackwood's Magazine. His first published piece, "The Mystery of Sasassa Valley", a story set in South Africa, was printed in Chambers's Edinburgh Journal on September 6, 1879. Later that month, on September 20, Sir Arthur Conan Doyle published his first non-fictional article, "Gelsemium as a Poison" in the British Medical Journal.

Following his term at the university, he was employed as a doctor on the Greenland whaler - the Hope of Peterhead in 1880 and after his graduation, as a ship's surgeon on the SS Mayumba during a voyage to the West African coast in 1881. He completed his doctorate on the subject of tabes dorsalis in 1885.

Literary Works and Achievements

His practice was initially not very successful. While waiting for patients, Conan Doyle again began writing stories and composed his first novels, *The Mystery of Cloomber*, not published until 1888, and the unfinished *Narrative of John Smith*, which went unpublished until 2011. He amassed a portfolio of short stories including "The Captain of the Pole-Star" and "J. Habakuk Jephson's Statement", both inspired by Doyle's time at sea.

Doyle struggled to find a publisher for his work. His first significant piece, *A Study in Scarlet*, was taken by Ward Lock & Co on November 20, 1886, giving Doyle £25 for all rights to the story. The piece appeared later that year in the Beeton's Christmas Annual and received good reviews in *The Scotsman and the Glasgow Herald*. The story featured the first appearance of Watson and Sherlock Holmes, partially modelled after his former university teacher, Joseph Bell.

Death of Sherlock Holmes

In December 1893, in order to dedicate more of his time to what he considered his more important works (his historical novels), Conan Doyle had Holmes and Professor Moriarty apparently plunge to their deaths together down the Reichenbach Falls in the story "The Final Problem". Public outcry, however, led him to bring the character back in 1901, in "The Hound of the Baskervilles", though this was set at a time before the Reichenbach incident. In 1903, Conan Doyle published his first Holmes short story in ten years, "The Adventure of the Empty House", in which it was explained that only Moriarty had fallen; but since Holmes had other dangerous enemies—especially, Colonel Sebastian Moran—he had arranged to also be perceived as dead. Holmes ultimately was featured in a total of **56 short stories** and **four Conan Doyle novels**, and has since appeared in many novels and stories by other authors too.

Later Years

Following the death of his wife, Louisa in 1906, the death of his son, Kingsley, just before the end of World War I, and the deaths of his brother, Innes, his two brothers-in-laws (one of whom was E. W. Hornung, creator of the literary character, Raffles) and his two nephews, shortly after the war, Conan Doyle sank into depression. He found solace supporting spiritualism and its attempts to find proof of existence beyond the grave. He was also a member of the renowned paranormal organisation, **The Ghost Club**. Its focus, then and now, is on the scientific study of alleged paranormal activities in order to prove (or refute) the existence of paranormal phenomena.

His book, *The Coming of the Fairies (1921)* shows he was apparently convinced of the veracity of the five Cottingley Fairies photographs (which decades later were exposed as a hoax). *In The History of Spiritualism* (1926), Conan Doyle praised the psychic phenomena and spirit materialisations produced by Eusapia Palladino and Mina "Margery" Crandon.

Sir Arthur Conan Doyle was found clutching his chest in the hall of Windlesham, his house in Crowborough, East Sussex, on July 7, 1930. He died of a heart attack at the age of 71. His grave is at Minstead, England.

Trivia

A statue honours Conan Doyle at Crowborough Cross in Crowborough, where he lived for 23 years. There is also a statue of Sherlock Holmes in Picardy Place, Edinburgh, close to the house, where Conan Doyle was born.

The Adventure of the Noble Bachelor

~ Arthur Conan Doyle

THe Lord St. Simons marriage, and its curious termination, have long ceased to be a subject of interest in those *exalted* circles in which the unfortunate bridegroom moves. Fresh scandals have eclipsed it, and their more *piquant* details have drawn the gossips away from this four-year-old drama. As I have reason to believe, however, that the full facts have never been revealed to the general public, and as my friend Sherlock Holmes had a considerable share in clearing the matter up, I feel that no *memoir* of him would be complete without some little sketch of this remarkable episode.

It was a few weeks before my own marriage, during the days when I was still sharing rooms with Holmes in Baker Street, that he came home from an afternoon stroll to find a letter on the table waiting for him. I had remained indoors all day, for the weather had taken a sudden turn to rain, with high autumnal winds, and the Jezail bullet which I had brought back in one of my limbs as a relic of my Afghan campaign throbbed with dull persistence. With my body in one easy-chair and my legs upon another, I had surrounded myself with a cloud of newspapers until at last, saturated with the news of the day, I tossed them all aside and lay listless, watching the huge *crest* and *monogram* upon the envelope upon the table and wondering lazily who my friend's noble correspondent could be.

"Here is a very fashionable *epistle*," I remarked as he entered. "Your morning letters, if I remember right, were from a fish-monger and a tide-waiter."

"Yes, my correspondence has certainly the charm of variety," he answered, smiling, "and the humbler are usually the more interesting. This looks like one of those unwelcome social summonses which call upon a man either to be bored or to lie."

He broke the seal and glanced over the contents.

"Oh, come, it may prove to be something of interest, after all."

Memoir - *A record of events*
Crest - *The head or top of anything*
Monogram - *An emblem*
Exalted – *Dignified*
Piquant – *Strong and sharp*

Greatest   Adventure   Stories   of   Sherloc

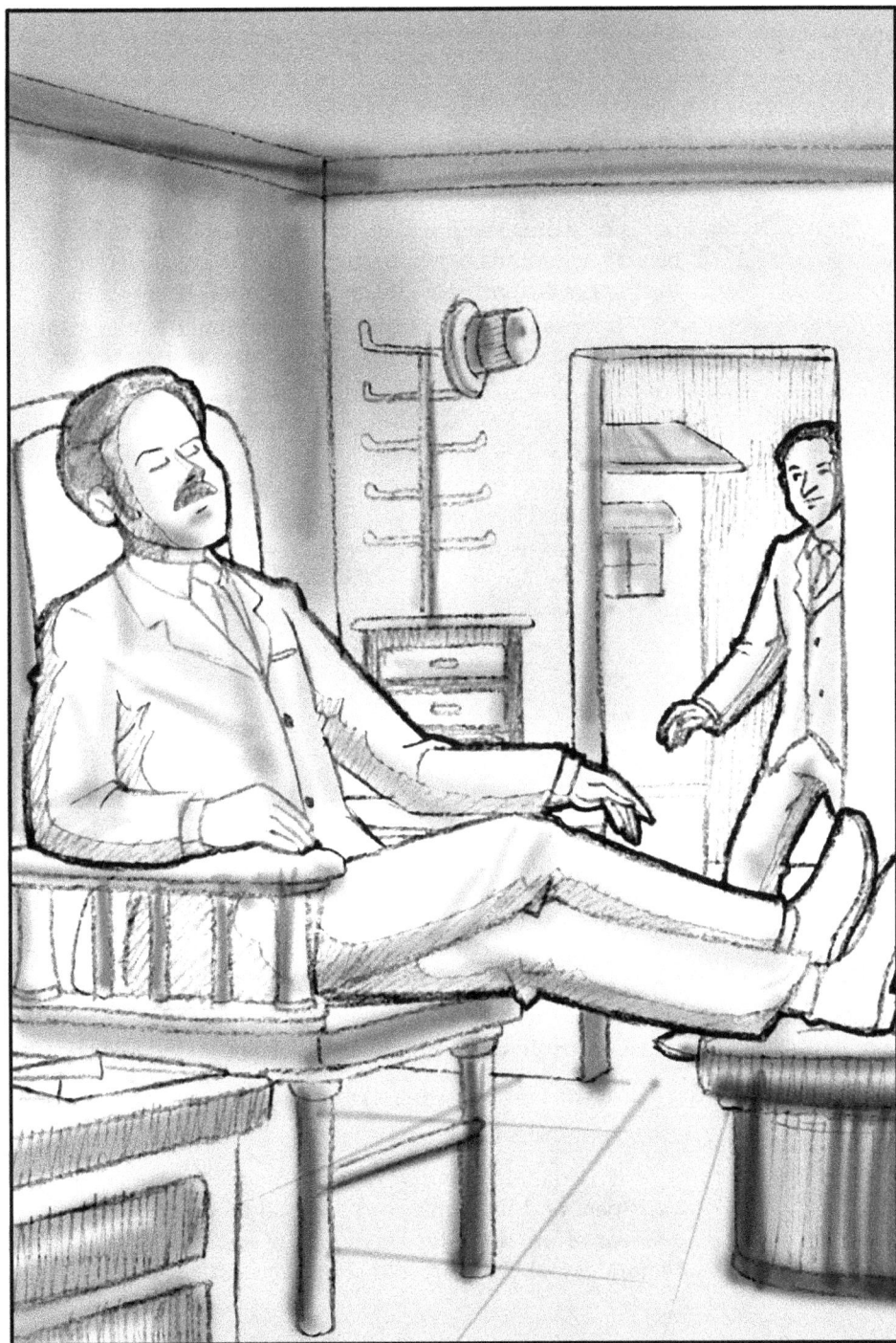

"Not social, then?"

"No, distinctly professional."

"And from a noble client?"

"One of the highest in England."

"My dear fellow, I congratulate you."

"I assure you, Watson, without affectation, that the status of my client is a matter of less moment to me than the interest of his case. It is just possible, however, that that also may not be wanting in this new investigation. You have been reading the papers *diligently* of late, have you not?"

"It looks like it," said I *ruefully*, pointing to a huge bundle in the corner. "I have had nothing else to do."

"It is fortunate, for you will perhaps be able to post me up. I read nothing except the criminal news and the agony column. The latter is always instructive. But if you have followed recent events so closely you must have read about Lord St. Simon and his wedding?"

"Oh, yes, with the deepest interest."

"That is well. The letter which I hold in my hand is from Lord St. Simon. I will read it to you, and in return, you must turn over these papers and let me have whatever bears upon the matter. This is what he says:

"'MY DEAR MR. SHERLOCK HOLMES,

"'Lord Backwater tells me that I may place implicit reliance upon your judgement and *discretion*. I have determined, therefore, to call upon you and to consult you in reference to the very painful event which has occurred in connection with my wedding. Mr. Lestrade, of Scotland Yard, is acting already in the matter, but he assures me that he sees no objection to your cooperation, and that he even thinks that it might be of some assistance. I will call at four o'clock in the afternoon, and, should you have any other engagement at that time, I hope that you will postpone it, as this matter is of *paramount* importance.

"'Yours faithfully,

"'ST. SIMON.'

"It is dated from Grosvenor Mansions, written with a *quill* pen, and the noble lord has had the misfortune to get a smear of ink upon the outer side of his right little finger," remarked Holmes as he folded up the *epistle*.

Diligently -
Persistently
Paramount - *Chief,*
Greatest, Atmost
Discretion - *Choice*
Ruefully –
Apologetically

Greatest   Adventure   Stories   of   Sherloc

"He says four o'clock. It is three now. He will be here in an hour."

"Then I have just time, with your assistance, to get clear upon the subject. Turn over those papers and arrange the extracts in their order of time, while I take a glance as to who our client is." He picked a red-covered volume from a line of books of reference beside the mantelpiece. "Here he is," said he, sitting down and flattening it out upon his knee. "Lord Robert Walsingham de Vere St. Simon, second son of the Duke of Balmoral. Hum! Arms: Azure, three *caltrops* in chief over a *fess sable*. Born in 1846. He's forty-one years of age, which is mature for marriage. Was Under-Secretary for the colonies in a late administration. The Duke, his father, was at one time Secretary for Foreign Affairs. They inherit Plantagenet blood by direct *descent*, and Tudor on the *distaff* side. Ha! Well, there is nothing very instructive in all this. I think that I must turn to you Watson, for something more solid."

"I have very little difficulty in finding what I want," said I, "for the facts are quite recent, and the matter struck me as remarkable. I feared to refer them to you, however, as I knew that you had an inquiry on hand and that you disliked the *intrusion* of other matters."

"Oh, you mean the little problem of the Grosvenor Square furniture van. That is quite cleared up now – though, indeed, it was obvious from the first. Pray give me the results of your newspaper selections."

"Here is the first notice which I can find. It is in the personal column of the Morning Post, and dates, as you see, some weeks back: 'A marriage has been arranged,' it says, 'and will, if rumour is correct, very shortly take place, between Lord Robert St. Simon, second son of the Duke of Balmoral, and Miss Hatty Doran, the only daughter of Aloysius Doran, Esq., of San Francisco, Cal., U.S.A.' That is all."

"Terse and to the point," remarked Holmes, stretching his long, thin legs towards the fire.

"There was a paragraph amplifying this in one of the society papers of the same week. Ah, here it is: 'There will soon be a call for protection in the marriage market, for the present free-trade principle appears to tell heavily against our home product. One by one the management of the noble houses of Great Britain is passing into the hands of our fair cousins from

Intrusion - *A wrongful entry*
Fess - *A broad horizontal band*
Sable - *A mourning garment*
Descent - *Action of moving downwards*
Caltrops – *An anti-personnel weapon made of two or more sharp nails*
Distaff – *A staff used in spinning*

across the Atlantic. An important addition has been made during the last week to the list of the prizes which have been borne away by these charming invaders. Lord St. Simon, who has shown himself for over twenty years proof against *the little god's arrows,* has now definitely announced his approaching marriage with Miss Hatty Doran, the fascinating daughter of a California millionaire. Miss Doran, whose graceful figure and striking face attracted much attention at the Westbury House festivities, is an only child, and it is currently reported that her dowry will run to considerably over the six figures, with expectancies for the future. As it is an open secret that the Duke of Balmoral has been compelled to sell his pictures within the last few years, and as Lord St. Simon has no property of his own save the small estate of Birchmoor, it is obvious that the Californian heiress is not the only gainer by an alliance which will enable her to make the easy and common transition from a Republican lady to a British *peeress.*'"

"Anything else?" asked Holmes, yawning.

"Oh, yes; plenty. Then there is another note in the Morning Post to say that the marriage would be an absolutely quiet one, that it would be at St. George's, Hanover Square, that only half a dozen intimate friends would be invited, and that the party would return to the furnished house at Lancaster Gate which has been taken by Mr. Aloysius Doran. Two days later – that is, on Wednesday last – there is a curt announcement that the wedding had taken place, and that the honeymoon would be passed at Lord Backwater's place, near Petersfield. Those are all the notices which appeared before the disappearance of the bride."

"Before the what?" asked Holmes with a start.

"The vanishing of the lady."

"When did she vanish, then?"

"At the wedding breakfast."

"Indeed. This is more interesting than it promised to be; quite dramatic, in fact."

"Yes; it struck me as being a little out of the common."

"They often vanish before the ceremony, and occasionally during the honeymoon; but I cannot call to mind anything quite so prompt as this. Pray let me have the details."

"I warn you that they are very incomplete."

"Perhaps, we may make them less so."

"Such as they are, they are set forth in a single article of a morning paper of yesterday, which I will read to you. It is headed, 'Singular Occurrence at a Fashionable Wedding':

"'The family of Lord Robert St. Simon has been thrown into the greatest *consternation* by the strange and painful episodes which have taken place in connection with his wedding. The ceremony, as shortly announced in the papers of yesterday, occurred on the previous morning; but it is only now that it has been possible to confirm the strange rumours which have been so persistently floating about. In spite of the attempts of the friends to hush the matter up, so much public attention has now been drawn to it that no good purpose can be served by affecting to disregard what is a common subject for conversation.

"'The ceremony, which was performed at St. George's, Hanover Square, was a very quiet one, no one being present save the father of the bride, Mr. Aloysius Doran, the Duchess of Balmoral, Lord Backwater, Lord Eustace, and Lady Clara St. Simon (the younger brother and sister of the bridegroom), and Lady Alicia Whittington. The whole party proceeded afterwards to the house of Mr. Aloysius Doran, at Lancaster Gate, where breakfast had been prepared. It appears that some little trouble was caused by a woman, whose name has not been ascertained, who endeavoured to force her way into the house after the bridal party, alleging that she had some claim upon Lord St. Simon. It was only after a painful and prolonged scene that she was *ejected* by the butler and the footman. The bride, who had fortunately entered the house before this unpleasant interruption, had sat down to breakfast with the rest, when she complained of a sudden *indisposition* and retired to her room. Her prolonged absence having caused some comment, her father followed her, but learned from her maid that she had only come up to her chamber for an instant, caught up an *ulster* and *bonnet*, and hurried down to the passage. One of the footmen declared that he had seen a lady leave the house thus apparelled, but had refused to credit that it was his mistress, believing her to be with the company. On ascertaining that his daughter had disappeared, Mr. Aloysius Doran, in conjunction with the bridegroom, instantly put themselves in communication with the police, and very energetic inquiries are being made, which will probably result in a speedy clearing up of this very singular business.

Ejected - *Thrown out*
Ulster - *Long loose overcoat*
Bonnet - *The ceremonial feathered headdress*
Consternation – *Anxiety, Dismay*
Indisposition – *Mild illness*

Up to a late hour last night, however, nothing had transpired as to the whereabouts of the missing lady. There are rumours of foul play in the matter, and it is said that the police have caused the arrest of the woman who had caused the original disturbance, in the belief that, from jealousy or some other motive, she may have been concerned in the strange disappearance of the bride.'"

"And is that all?"

"Only one little item in another of the morning papers, but it is a suggestive one."

"And it is –"

"That Miss Flora Millar, the lady who had caused the disturbance, has actually been arrested. It appears that she was formerly a *danseuse* at the Allegro, and that she has known the bridegroom for some years. There are no further particulars, and the whole case is in your hands now – so far as it has been set forth in the public press."

"And an exceedingly interesting case it appears to be. I would not have missed it for worlds. But there is a ring at the bell, Watson, and as the clock makes it a few minutes after four, I have no doubt that this will prove to be our noble client. Do not dream of going, Watson, for I very much prefer having a witness, if only as a check to my own memory."

"Lord Robert St. Simon," announced our page-boy, throwing open the door. A gentleman entered, with a pleasant, cultured face, high-nosed and pale, with something perhaps of *petulance* about the mouth, and with the steady, well-opened eye of a man whose pleasant lot it had ever been to command and to be obeyed. His manner was *brisk*, and yet his general appearance gave an undue impression of age, for he had a slight forward stoop and a little bend of the knees as he walked. His hair, too, as he swept off his very curly-brimmed hat, was *grizzled* around the edges and thin upon the top. As to his dress, it was careful to the verge of *foppishness*, with high collar, black frock-coat, white waistcoat, yellow gloves, patent-leather shoes, and light-coloured *gaiters*. He advanced slowly into the room, turning his head from left to right, and swinging in his right hand the cord which held his golden eyeglasses.

"Good-day, Lord St. Simon," said Holmes, rising and bowing. "Pray take the basket-chair. This is my friend and colleague, Dr. Watson. Draw up a little to the fire, and we will talk this matter over."

Gaiters - *A garment similar to leggings*
Brisk - *Active, fast and energetic*
Grizzled - *Streaked with grey hair*
Danseuse – *A ballet dancer*
Petulance – *Bad temper*

Greatest   Adventure   Stories   of   Sherloc

"A most painful matter to me, as you can most readily imagine, Mr. Holmes. I have been **cut to the quick.** I understand that you have already managed several delicate cases of this sort sir, though I presume that they were hardly from the same class of society."

"No, I am descending."

"I beg pardon."

"My last client of the sort was a king."

"Oh, really! I had no idea. And which king?"

"The King of Scandinavia."

"What! Had he lost his wife?"

"You can understand," said Holmes *suavely*, "that I extend to the affairs of my other clients the same secrecy which I promise to you in yours."

"Of course! Very right! very right! I'm sure I beg pardon. As to my own case, I am ready to give you any information which may assist you in forming an opinion."

"Thank you. I have already learned all that is in the public prints, nothing more. I presume that I may take it as correct–this article, for example, as to the disappearance of the bride."

Lord St. Simon glanced over it. "Yes, it is correct, as far as it goes."

"But it needs a great deal of *supplementing* before anyone could offer an opinion. I think that I may arrive at my facts most directly by questioning you."

"Pray do so."

"When did you first meet Miss Hatty Doran?"

"In San Francisco, a year ago."

"You were travelling in the States?"

"Yes."

"Did you become engaged then?"

"No."

"But you were on a friendly footing?"

"I was amused by her society, and she could see that I was amused."

"Her father is very rich?"

"He is said to be the richest man on the Pacific slope."

"And how did he make his money?"

Suavely - *In a charming manner*
Cut to the quick – *To upset someone by criticising them*
Supplementing – *Adding*

"In mining. He had nothing a few years ago. Then he struck gold, invested it, and came up by leaps and bounds."

"Now, what is your own impression as to the young lady's – your wife's character?"

The nobleman swung his glasses a little faster and stared down into the fire. "You see, Mr. Holmes," said he, "my wife was twenty before her father became a rich man. During that time she ran free in a mining camp and wandered through, woods or mountains, so that her education has come from Nature rather than from the schoolmaster. She is what we call in England a tomboy, with a strong nature, wild and free, *unfettered* by any sort of traditions. She is *impetuous* – volcanic, I was about to say. She is swift in making up her mind and fearless in carrying out her resolutions. On the other hand, I would not have given her the name which I have the honour to bear" – he gave a little stately cough – "had not I thought her to be at bottom a noble woman. I believe that she is capable of heroic self-sacrifice and that anything dishonourable would be *repugnant* to her."

"Have you her photograph?"

"I brought this with me." He opened a locket and showed us the full face of a very lovely woman. It was not a photograph but an ivory miniature, and the artist had brought out the full effect of the lustrous black hair, the large dark eyes, and the exquisite mouth. Holmes gazed long and earnestly at it. Then he closed the locket and handed it back to Lord St. Simon. "The young lady came to London, then, and you renewed your acquaintance?"

"Yes, her father brought her over for this last London season. I met her several times, became engaged to her, and have now married her."

"She brought, I understand, a considerable dowry?"

"A fair dowry. Not more than is usual in my family."

"And this, of course, remains to you, since the marriage is *a fait accompli?*"

"I really have made no inquiries on the subject."

"Very naturally not. Did you see Miss Doran on the day before the wedding?"

"Yes."

"Was she in good spirits?"

Impetuous –
Impulsive
A fait accompli –
Accomplished or
established fact

Greatest   Adventure   Stories   of   Sherloc

"Never better. She kept talking of what we should do in our future lives."

"Indeed! That is very interesting. And on the morning of the wedding?"

"She was as bright as possible – at least until after the ceremony."

"And did you observe any change in her then?"

"Well, to tell the truth, I saw then the first signs that I had ever seen that her temper was just a little sharp. The incident however, was too trivial to relate and can have no possible bearing upon the case."

"Pray let us have it, for all that."

"Oh, it is childish. She dropped her bouquet as we went towards the *vestry*. She was passing the front *pew* at the time, and it fell over into the pew. There was a moment's delay, but the gentleman in the pew handed it up to her again, and it did not appear to be the worse for the fall. Yet when I spoke to her of the matter, she answered me abruptly; and in the carriage, on our way home, she seemed absurdly agitated over this trifling cause."

"Indeed! You say that there was a gentleman in the pew. Some of the general public were present, then?"

"Oh, yes. It is impossible to exclude them when the church is open."

"This gentleman was not one of your wife's friends?"

"No, no; I call him a gentleman by courtesy, but he was quite a common-looking person. I hardly noticed his appearance. But really I think that we are wandering rather far from the point."

"Lady St. Simon, then, returned from the wedding in a less cheerful frame of mind than she had gone to it. What did she do on re-entering her father's house?"

"I saw her in conversation with her maid."

"And who is her maid?"

"Alice is her name. She is an American and came from California with her."

"A *confidential* servant?"

"A little too much so. It seemed to me that her mistress allowed her to take great liberties. Still, of course, in America they look upon these things in a different way."

Confidential - *Private or secret*
Vestry – *A room attached to a church, used for record-keeping, etc.*
Pew – *A long bench with a back*

"How long did she speak to the Alice?"

"Oh, a few minutes. I had something else to think of."

"You did not overhear what they said?"

"Lady St. Simon said something about 'jumping a claim.' She was accustomed to use **slang** of the kind. I have no idea what she meant."

"American slang is very expressive sometimes. And what did your wife do when she finished speaking to her maid?"

"She walked into the breakfast-room."

"On your arm?"

"No, alone. She was very independent in little matters like that. Then, after we had sat down for ten minutes or so, she rose hurriedly, muttered some words of apology, and left the room. She never came back."

"But this maid, Alice, as I understand, **deposes** that she went to her room, covered her bride's dress with a long ulster, put on a bonnet, and went out."

"Quite so. And she was afterwards seen walking into Hyde Park in company with Flora Millar, a woman who is now in custody, and who had already made a disturbance at Mr. Doran's house that morning."

"Ah, yes. I should like a few particulars as to this young lady, and your relations to her."

Lord St. Simon shrugged his shoulders and raised his eyebrows. "We have been on a friendly footing for some years – I may say on a very friendly footing. She used to be at the Allegro. I have not treated her ungenerously, and she had no just cause of complaint against me, but you know what women are, Mr. Holmes. Flora was a dear little thing, but exceedingly hot-headed and devotedly attached to me. She wrote me dreadful letters when she heard that I was about to be married, and, to tell the truth, the reason why I had the marriage celebrated so quietly was that I feared lest there might be a scandal in the church. She came to Mr. Doran's door just after we returned, and she endeavoured to push her way in, uttering very abusive expressions towards my wife, and even threatening her, but I had foreseen the possibility of something of the sort, and I had two police fellows there in private clothes, who soon pushed her out again. She was quiet when she saw that there was no good in making a row."

"Did your wife hear all this?"

Slang – *Colloquial speech*
Deposes – *Removes*

"No, thank goodness, she did not."

"And she was seen walking with this very woman afterwards?"

"Yes. That is what Mr. Lestrade, of Scotland Yard, looks upon as so serious. It is thought that Flora *decoyed* my wife out and laid some terrible trap for her."

"Well, it is a possible *supposition*."

"You think so, too?"

"I did not say a probable one. But you do not yourself look upon this as likely?"

"I do not think Flora would hurt a fly."

"Still, jealousy is a strange transformer of characters. Pray what is your own theory as to what took place?"

"Well, really, I came to seek a theory, not to propound one. I have given you all the facts. Since you ask me, however, I may say that it has occurred to me as possible that the excitement of this affair, the consciousness that she had made so immense a social *stride*, had the effect of causing some little nervous disturbance in my wife."

"In short, that she had become suddenly *deranged*?"

"Well, really, when I consider that she has turned her back – I will not say upon me, but upon so much that many have aspired to without success – I can hardly explain it in any other fashion."

"Well, certainly that is also a *conceivable* hypothesis," said Holmes, smiling. "And now, Lord St. Simon, I think that I have nearly all my data. May I ask whether you were seated at the breakfast-table so that you could see out of the window?"

"We could see the other side of the road and the Park."

"Quite so. Then I do not think that I need to detain you longer. I shall communicate with you." "Should you be fortunate enough to solve this problem," said our client, rising.

"I have solved it."

"Eh? What was that?"

"I say that I have solved it."

"Where, then, is my wife?"

"That is a detail which I shall speedily supply."

Lord St. Simon shook his head. "I am afraid that it will take wiser heads than yours or mine," he remarked, and bowing in a stately, old-fashioned manner he departed.

Conceivable - *Thinkable, Possible*
Decoyed – *Tricked*
Deranged – *Crazy*

"It is very good of Lord St. Simon to honour my head by putting it on a level with his own," said Sherlock Holmes, laughing. "I think that I shall have a whisky and soda and a cigar after all this cross-questioning. I had formed my conclusions as to the case before our client came into the room."

"My dear Holmes!"

"I have notes of several similar cases, though none, as I remarked before, which were quite as prompt. My whole examination served to turn my **conjecture** into a certainty. Circumstantial evidence is occasionally very convincing, as when you find a **trout** in the milk, to quote Thoreau's example."

"But I have heard all that you have heard."

"Without, however, the knowledge of pre-existing cases which serves me so well. There was a parallel instance in Aberdeen some years back, and something on very much the same lines at Munich the year after the Franco-Prussian War. It is one of these cases – but, hello, here is Lestrade! Good-afternoon, Lestrade! You will find an extra tumbler upon the sideboard, and there are cigars in the box."

The official detective was attired in a pea-jacket and *cravat*, which gave him a decidedly nautical appearance, and he carried a black canvas bag in his hand. With a short greeting, he seated himself and lit the cigar which had been offered to him.

"What's up, then?" asked Holmes with a twinkle in his eye. "You look dissatisfied."

"And I feel dissatisfied. It is this **infernal** St. Simon marriage case. I can make neither head nor tail of the business."

"Really! You surprise me."

"Whoever heard of such a mixed affair? Every clue seems to slip through my fingers. I have been at work upon it all day."

"And very wet it seems to have made you," said Holmes laying his hand upon the arm of the pea-jacket.

"Yes, I have been dragging the Serpentine."

"In heaven's name, what for?"

"In search of the body of Lady St. Simon."

Sherlock Holmes leaned back in his chair and laughed heartily.

Conjecture - *An opinion or conclusion*
Cravat - *A strip of fabric worn around the neck*
Trout – *A freshwater fish*
Infernal – *Hellish*

"Have you dragged the basin of Trafalgar Square fountain?" he asked.

"Why? What do you mean?"

"Because you have just as good a chance of finding this lady in the one as in the other."

Lestrade shot an angry glance at my companion. "I suppose you know all about it," he **snarled**. "Well, I have only just heard the facts, but my mind is made up."

"Oh, indeed! Then you think that the Serpentine plays no part in the maner?"

"I think it very unlikely."

"Then perhaps you will kindly explain how it is that we found this in it?" He opened his bag as he spoke, and tumbled onto the floor a wedding-dress of watered silk, a pair of white satin shoes and a bride's **wreath** and veil, all discoloured and soaked in water. "There," said he, putting a new wedding-ring upon the top of the pile. "There is a little nut for you to crack, Master Holmes."

"Oh, indeed!" said my friend, blowing blue rings into the air. "You dragged them from the Serpentine?"

"No. They were found floating near the margin by a park-keeper. They have been identified as her clothes, and it seemed to me that if the clothes were there the body would not be far off."

"By the same brilliant reasoning, every man's body is to be found in the neighbourhood of his wardrobe. And pray what did you hope to arrive at through this?"

"At some evidence **implicating** Flora Millar in the disappearance."

"I am afraid that you will find it difficult."

"Are you, indeed, now?" cried Lestrade with some bitterness. "I am afraid, Holmes, that you are not very practical with your deductions and your inferences. You have made two blunders in as many minutes. This dress does implicate Miss Flora Millar."

"And how?"

"In the dress is a pocket. In the pocket is a card-case. In the card-case is a note. And here is the very note." He slapped it down upon the table in front of him. "Listen to this: 'You will see me when all is ready. Come at once. F.H.M.' Now my theory

Wreath - *An arrangement of flowers*
Implicating – *Accusing*
Snarled – *Growled*

all along has been that Lady St. Simon was decoyed away by Flora Millar, and that she, with *confederates*, no doubt, was responsible for her disappearance. Here, signed with her initials, is the very note which was no doubt quietly slipped into her hand at the door and which lured her within their reach."

"Very good, Lestrade," said Holmes, laughing. "You really are very fine indeed. Let me see it." He took up the paper in a listless way, but his attention instantly became *riveted*, and he gave a little cry of satisfaction. "This is indeed important," said he.

"Ha! you find it so?"

"Extremely so. I congratulate you warmly."

Lestrade rose in his triumph and bent his head to look. "Why," he shrieked, "you're looking at the wrong side!"

"On the contrary, this is the right side."

"The right side? You're mad! Here is the note written in pencil over here."

"And over here is what appears to be the fragment of a hotel bill, which interests me deeply."

"There's nothing in it. I looked at it before," said Lestrade. "'Oct. 4th, rooms 8s., breakfast 2s. 6d., cocktail 1s., lunch 2s. 6d., glass sherry, 8d.' I see nothing in that."

"Very likely not. It is most important, all the same. As to the note, it is important also, or at least the initials are, so I congratulate you again."

"I've wasted time enough," said Lestrade, rising. "I believe in hard work and not in sitting by the fire spinning fine theories. Good-day, Mr. Holmes, and we shall see which gets to the bottom of the matter first." He gathered up the garments, thrust them into the bag, and made for the door.

"Just one hint to you, Lestrade," *drawled* Holmes before his rival vanished; "I will tell you the true solution of the matter. Lady St. Simon is a myth. There is not, and there never has been, any such person."

Lestrade looked sadly at my companion. Then he turned to me, tapped his forehead three times, shook his head solemnly, and hurried away.

He had hardly shut the door behind him when Holmes rose to put on his overcoat. "There is something in what the

Riveted - Joined or fastened
Confederates – *Partners*
Drawled – *Spoke lazily with lengthened vowels*

Greatest   Adventure   Stories   of   Sherloc

fellow says about outdoor work," he remarked, "so I think, Watson, that I must leave you to your papers for a little."

It was after five o'clock when Sherlock Holmes left me, but I had no time to be lonely, for within an hour, there arrived a confectioner's man with a very large flat box. This he unpacked with the help of a youth whom he had brought with him, and presently, to my very great astonishment, a quite *epicurean* little cold supper began to be laid out upon our humble lodging-house mahogany.

There were a couple of *brace* of cold woodcock, a *pheasant*, a pate de foie gras pie with a group of ancient and cobwebby bottles. Having laid out all these luxuries, my two visitors vanished away, like the genii of the Arabian Nights, with no explanation save that the things had been paid for and were ordered to this address.

Just before nine o'clock, Sherlock Holmes stepped briskly into the room. His features were gravely set, but there was a light in his eye which made me think that he had not been disappointed in his conclusions.

"They have laid the supper, then," he said, rubbing his hands.

"You seem to expect company. They have laid for five."

"Yes, I fancy we may have some company dropping in," said he. "I am surprised that Lord St. Simon has not already arrived. Ha! I fancy that I hear his step now upon the stairs."

It was indeed our visitor of the afternoon who came bustling in, dangling his glasses more vigorously than ever, and with a very perturbed expression upon his aristocratic features.

"My messenger reached you, then?" asked Holmes.

"Yes, and I confess that the contents startled me beyond measure. Have you good authority for what you say?"

"The best possible."

Lord St. Simon sank into a chair and passed his hand over his forehead.

"What will the Duke say," he murmured, "when he hears that one of the family has been subjected to such humiliation?"

"It is the purest accident. I cannot allow that there is any humiliation."

Pheasant - *A large, long tailed game bird*

Epicurean – *Luxurious*

Brace – *Group*

"Ah, you look on these things from another standpoint."

"I fail to see that anyone is to blame. I can hardly see how the lady could have acted otherwise, though her abrupt method of doing it was undoubtedly to be regretted. Having no mother, she had no one to advise her at such a crisis."

"It was a *slight*, sir, a public slight," said Lord St. Simon, tapping his fingers upon the table. "You must make allowance for this poor girl, placed in so *unprecedented* a position."

"I will make no allowance. I am very angry indeed, and I have been shamefully used."

"I think that I heard a ring," said Holmes. "Yes, there are steps on the landing. If I cannot persuade you to take a lenient view of the matter, Lord St. Simon, I have brought an advocate here who may be more successful."

He opened the door and ushered in a lady and gentleman. "Lord St. Simon," said he "allow me to introduce you to Mr. and Mrs. Francis Hay Moulton. The lady, I think, you have already met."

At the sight of these newcomers, our client had sprung from his seat and stood very erect, with his eyes cast down and his hand thrust into the breast of his frock-coat, a picture of offended dignity. The lady had taken a quick step forward and had held out her hand to him, but he still refused to raise his eyes. It was as well for his resolution, perhaps, for her pleading face was one which it was hard to resist.

"You're angry, Robert," said she. "Well, I guess you have every cause to be."

"Pray make no apology to me," said Lord St. Simon bitterly.

"Oh, yes, I know that I have treated you real bad and that I should have spoken to you before I went; but I was kind of *rattled*, and from the time when I saw Frank here again I just didn't know what I was doing or saying. I only wonder I didn't fall down and do a faint right there before the *altar*."

"Perhaps, Mrs. Moulton, you would like my friend and me to leave the room while you explain this matter?"

"If I may give an opinion," remarked the strange gentleman, "we've had just a little too much secrecy over this business already. For my part, I should like all Europe and America

Petered - *Decrease or fade*
Altar - *Table or flat block*
Unprecedented - *Unparalleled*
Rattled - *Make a rapid succession of short, sharp sounds*
Slight – *Insult*
Wiry – *Thin*

to hear the rights of it." He was a small, **wiry**, sunburnt man, clean-shaven, with a sharp face and alert manner.

"Then I'll tell our story right away," said the lady. "Frank here and I met in '84, in McQuire's camp, near the Rockies, where pa was working a claim. We were engaged to each other, Frank and I; but then one day father struck a rich pocket and made a pile, while poor Frank here had a claim that *petered* out and came to nothing.

The richer pa grew, the poorer was Frank; so at last pa wouldn't hear of our engagement lasting any longer, and he took me away to 'Frisco. Frank wouldn't throw up his hand, though; so he followed me there, and he saw me without pa knowing anything about it. It would only have made him mad to know, so we just fixed it all up for ourselves. Frank said that he would go and make his pile, too, and never come back to claim me until he had as much as pa.

So then I promised to wait for him to the end of time and pledged myself not to marry anyone else while he lived. 'Why shouldn't we be married right away, then,' said he, 'and then I will feel sure of you; and I won't claim to be your husband until I come back?' Well, we talked it over, and he had fixed it all up so nicely, with a clergyman all ready in waiting, that we just did it right there; and then Frank went off to seek his fortune, and I went back to pa.

"The next I heard of Frank was that he was in Montana, and then he went *prospecting* in Arizona, and then I heard of him from New Mexico. After that came a long newspaper story about how a miners' camp had been attacked by *Apache Indians*, and there was my Frank's name among the killed.

I fainted dead away, and I was very sick for months after. Pa thought I had a decline and took me to half the doctors in 'Frisco. Not a word of news came for a year and more, so that I never doubted that Frank was really dead. Then Lord St. Simon came to 'Frisco, and we came to London, and a marriage was arranged, and pa was very pleased, but I felt all the time that no man on this earth would ever take the place in my heart that had been given to my poor Frank.

"Still, if I had married Lord St. Simon, of course I'd have done my duty by him. We can't command our love, but we

Service - *Prayer*
Pew - *A long bench with a back placed in rows*
Prospecting – *Searching*
Apache Indians – *Groups of Native Americans*

can our actions. I went to the altar with him with the intention to make him just as good a wife as it was in me to be. But you may imagine what I felt when, just as I came to the altar rails, I glanced back and saw Frank standing and looking at me out of the first *pew*. I thought it was his ghost at first; but when I looked again there he was still, with a kind of question in his eyes, as if to ask me whether I were glad or sorry to see him. I wonder I didn't drop. I know that everything was turning around, and the words of the clergyman were just like the buzz of a bee in my ear.

I didn't know what to do. Should I stop the **service** and make a scene in the church? I glanced at him again, and he seemed to know what I was thinking, for he raised his finger to his lips to tell me to be still. Then I saw him scribble on a piece of paper, and I knew that he was writing me a note. As I passed his pew on the way out I dropped my bouquet over to him, and he slipped the note into my hand when he returned me the flowers.

It was only a line asking me to join him when he made the sign to me to do so. Of course, I never doubted for a moment that my first duty was now to him, and I determined to do just whatever he might direct.

"When I got back I told my maid, who had known him in California, and had always been his friend. I ordered her to say nothing, but to get a few things packed and my *ulster* ready. I know I ought to have spoken to Lord St. Simon, but it was **dreadful** hard before his mother and all those great people.

I just made up my mind to run away and explain afterwards. I hadn't been at the table ten minutes before I saw Frank out of the window at the other side of the road. He **beckoned** to me and then began walking into the Park. I slipped out, put on my things, and followed him. Some woman came talking something or other about Lord St. Simon to me – seemed to me from the little I heard as if he had a little secret of his own before marriage also – but I managed to get away from her and soon overtook Frank.

We got into a cab together, and away we drove to some lodgings he had taken in Gordon Square, and that was my true wedding after all those years of waiting. Frank had

Dreadfully - *Extremely*
Beckoned - *Make a gesture with the hand*
Ulster – *A long and loose overcoat worn by men*

been a prisoner among the Apaches, had escaped, came on to 'Frisco, found that I had given him up for dead and had gone to England, followed me there, and had come upon me at last on the very morning of my second wedding."

"I saw it in a paper," explained the American. "It gave the name and the church but not where the lady lived."

"Then we had a talk as to what we should do, and Frank was all for openness, but I was so ashamed of it all that I felt as if I should like to vanish away and never see any of them again – just sending a line for pa, perhaps, to show him that I was alive.

It was awful to me to think of all those lords and ladies sitting around that breakfast-table and waiting for me to come back. So Frank took my wedding-clothes and things and made a bundle of them, so that I should not be traced, and dropped them away somewhere where no one could find them.

It is likely that we should have gone on to Paris tomorrow, only that this good gentleman, Mr. Holmes, came around to us this evening, though how he found us is more than I can think, and he showed us very clearly and kindly that I was wrong and that Frank was right, and that we should be putting ourselves in the wrong if we were so secret.

Then he offered to give us a chance of talking to Lord St. Simon alone, and so we came right away around to his rooms at once. Now, Robert, you have heard it all, and I am very sorry if I have given you pain, and I hope that you do not think very meanly of me."

Lord St. Simon had by no means relaxed his rigid attitude, but had listened with a frowning brow and a compressed lip to this long narrative.

"Excuse me," he said, "but it is not my custom to discuss my most intimate personal affairs in this public manner."

"Then you won't forgive me? You won't shake hands before I go?"

"Oh, certainly, if it would give you any pleasure." He put out his hand and coldly grasped that which she extended to him.

"I had hoped," suggested Holmes, "that you would have joined us in a friendly supper."

In explicable - *Unable to be explained*

Acquie – *Agree*

Quartering – *Accommodating*

"I think that there you ask a little too much," responded his Lordship. "I may be forced to **acquiesce** in these recent developments, but I can hardly be expected to make merry over them. I think that with your permission I will now wish you all a very good-night." He included us all in a sweeping bow and stalked out of the room.

"Then I trust that you at least will honour me with your company," said Sherlock Holmes. "It is always a joy to meet an American, Mr. Moulton, for I am one of those who believe that the folly of a monarch and the blundering of a minister in far-gone years will not prevent our children from being some day citizens of the same world-wide country under a flag which shall be a **quartering** of the Union Jack with the Stars and Stripes."

"The case has been an interesting one," remarked Holmes when our visitors had left us, "because it serves to show very clearly how simple the **explanation** may be of an affair which at first sight seems to be almost inexplicable. Nothing could be more natural than the sequence of events as narrated by this lady, and nothing stranger than the result when viewed, for instance by Mr. Lestrade, of Scotland Yard."

"You were not yourself at fault at all, then?"

"From the first, two facts were very obvious to me, the one that the lady had been quite willing to undergo the wedding ceremony, the other that she had repented of it within a few minutes of returning home. Obviously something had occurred during the morning, then, to cause her to change her mind. What could that something be?

She could not have spoken to anyone when she was out, for she had been in the company of the bridegroom. Had she seen someone, then? If she had, it must be someone from America because she had spent so short a time in this country that she could hardly have allowed anyone to acquire so deep an influence over her that the mere sight of him would induce her to change her plans so completely.

You see we have already arrived, by a process of exclusion, at the idea that she might have seen an American. Then who could this American be, and why should he possess so much influence over her? It might be a lover; it might be a

Deduce - *Arrive at a conclusive, Result*
Parlance - *A particular way of speaking or using words*
Transparent – *Obvious, clear*
Allusion – *Reference*

husband. Her young womanhood had, I knew, been spent in rough scenes and under strange conditions.

So far I had got before I ever heard Lord St. Simon's narrative. When he told us of a man in a pew, of the change in the bride's manner, of so *transparent* a device for obtaining a note as the dropping of a bouquet, of her resort to her confidential maid, and of her very significant *allusion* to claim-jumping – which in miners' *parlance* means taking possession of that which another person has a prior claim to – the whole situation became absolutely clear. She had gone off with a man, and the man was either a lover or was a previous husband – the chances being in favour of the latter."

"And how in the world did you find them?"

"It might have been difficult, but friend Lestrade held information in his hands the value of which he did not himself know. The initials were, of course, of the highest importance, but more valuable still was it to know that within a week, he had settled his bill at one of the most select London hotels."

"How did you *deduce* the select?"

"By the select prices. Eight shillings for a bed and eightpence for a glass of sherry pointed to one of the most expensive hotels. There are not many in London which charge at that rate. In the second one which I visited in Northumberland Avenue, I learned by an inspection of the book that Francis H. Moulton, an American gentleman, had left only the day before, and on looking over the entries against him, I came upon the very items which I had seen in the duplicate bill.

His letters were to be forwarded to 226 Gordon Square; so *thither* I travelled, and being fortunate enough to find the loving couple at home, I *ventured* to give them some paternal advice and to point out to them that it would be better in every way that they should make their position a little clearer both to the general public and to Lord St. Simon in particular. I invited them to meet him here, and, as you see, I made him keep the appointment."

"But with no very good result," I remarked. "His conduct was certainly not very gracious."

Gracious - *Courteous, Kind*
Ventured - *Dared to do something*
Thither – *There*
Bleak – *Depressing*

"Ah, Watson," said Holmes, smiling, "perhaps you would not be very *gracious* either, if, after all the trouble of wooing and wedding, you found yourself deprived in an instant of wife and of fortune. I think that we may judge Lord St. Simon very mercifully and thank our stars that we are never likely to find ourselves in the same position. Draw your chair up and hand me my violin, for the only problem we have still to solve is how to while away these *bleak* autumnal evenings."

Food For Thought

If Lord St. Simon's wife had not seen Frank standing and looking at her from the first pew of the altar rails, what would have happened? What was her relation with Frank?

An Understanding

Q. 1. The Lord, St. Simon's marriage, and its curious termination was a subject of great interest in the dignified circles of Britain for long. Why was it so?

Ans. _____

_____

_____

_____

_____

Q. 2. How did the bride, Miss Doran disappear after her marriage just before the honeymoon?

Ans. _____

_____

_____

_____

Q. 3. "He is said to be the richest man on the Pacific slope." Who said these words to whom? How did Miss Doran's father make money?

Ans. _____

_____

_____

_____

Q. 4. Who was Flora Millar? What role did she play in the disappearance of Lord St. Simon's wife?

Ans. _____

_____

_____

_____

The Adventure of the Missing Three Quarter

~Arthur Conan Doyle

WE were fairly accustomed to receive weird telegrams at Baker Street, but I have a particular recollection of one which reached us on a gloomy February morning, some seven or eight years ago, and gave Mr. Sherlock Holmes a puzzled quarter of an hour. It was addressed to him, and ran thus:

Please await me. Terrible misfortune. Right wing three-quarter missing, indispensable tomorrow. OVERTON.

"Strand postmark, and dispatched ten thirty-six," said Holmes, reading it over and over. "Mr. Overton was evidently considerably excited when he sent it, and somewhat incoherent in consequence. Well, well, he will be here, I daresay, by the time I have looked through the TIMES, and then we shall know all about it. Even the most insignificant problem would be welcome in these stagnant days."

Things had indeed been very slow with us, and I had learned to dread such periods of inaction, for I knew by experience that my companion's brain was so abnormally active that it was dangerous to leave it without material upon which to work. For years, I had gradually *weaned* him from that drug mania which had threatened once to check his remarkable career. Now I knew that under ordinary conditions he no longer craved for this artificial *stimulus*, but I was well aware that the *fiend* was not dead but sleeping, and I have known that the sleep was a light one and the waking near when in periods of idleness, I have seen the drawn look upon Holmes's ascetic face, and the brooding of his deep-set and *inscrutable* eyes. Therefore I blessed this Mr. Overton whoever he might be, since he had come with his enigmatic message to break that dangerous calm which brought more peril to my friend than all the storms of his tempestuous life.

Fiend - *Evil spirit*
Inscrutable - *Impossible to understand*
Weaned – *Detached*
Stimulus – *Motivation*

As we had expected, the telegram was soon followed by its sender, and the card of Mr. Cyril Overton, Trinity College, Cambridge, announced the arrival of an enormous young man, sixteen stone of solid bone and muscle, who spanned

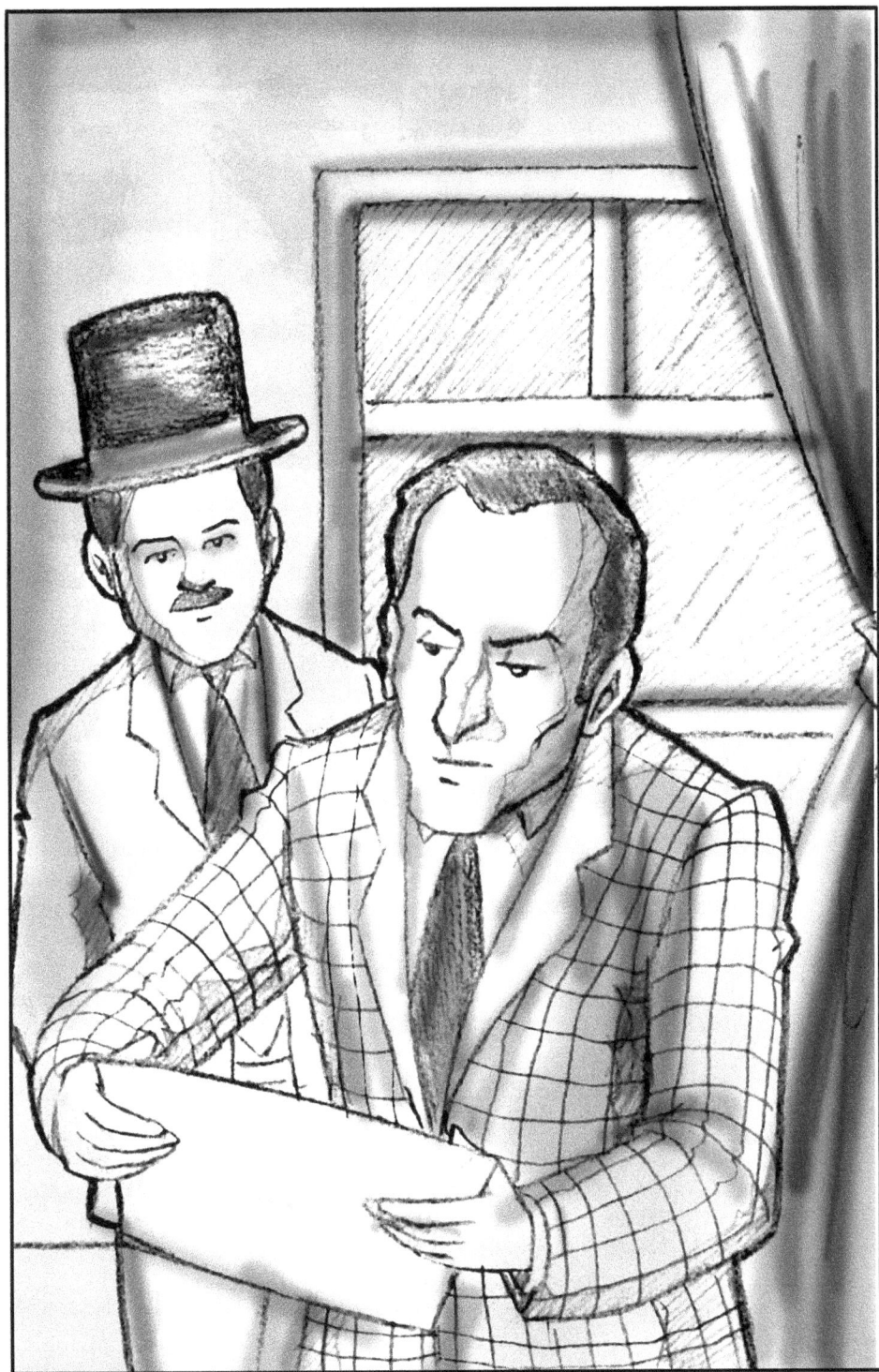

the doorway with his broad shoulders, and looked from one of us to the other with a *comely* face which was *haggard* with anxiety.

"Mr. Sherlock Holmes?"

My companion bowed.

"I've been down to Scotland Yard, Mr. Holmes. I saw Inspector Stanley Hopkins. He advised me to come to you. He said the case, so far as he could see, was more in your line than in that of the regular police."

"Pray sit down and tell me what is the matter."

"It's awful, Mr. Holmes – simply awful I wonder my hair isn't grey. Godfrey Staunton – you've heard of him, of course? He's simply the *hinge* that the whole team turns on. I'd rather spare two from the pack, and have Godfrey for my three-quarter line. Whether it's passing, or tackling, or *dribbling*, there's no one to touch him, and then, he's got the head, and can hold us all together. What am I to do? That's what I ask you, Mr. Holmes. There's Moorhouse, first reserve, but he is trained as a half, and he always edges right in on to the *scrum* instead of keeping out on the touchline. He's a fine place-kick, it's true, but then he has no judgement, and he can't *sprint* for nuts. Why, Morton or Johnson, the Oxford fliers, could *romp* round him. Stevenson is fast enough, but he couldn't drop from the twenty-five line, and a three-quarter who can't either *punt* or drop isn't worth a place for pace alone. No, Mr. Holmes, we are done unless you can help me to find Godfrey Staunton."

My friend had listened with amused surprise to this long speech, which was poured forth with extraordinary vigour and earnestness, every point being driven home by the slapping of a brawny hand upon the speaker's knee. When our visitor was silent, Holmes stretched out his hand and took down letter, "S" of his commonplace book. For once, he dug in vain into that mine of varied information.

Dribbling - *Trickle*
Hinge - *Part or a door/gate*
Comely - *Pleasant to look at*
Forger - *To imitate*
Haggard – *Tired*
Scrum – *A kind of formation of players on the field*

"There is Arthur H. Staunton, the rising young *forger*," said he, "and there was Henry Staunton, whom I helped to hang, but Godfrey Staunton is a new name to me."

It was our visitor's turn to look surprised.

"Why, Mr. Holmes, I thought you knew things," said he. "I suppose, then, if you have never heard of Godfrey Staunton, you don't know Cyril Overton either?"

Holmes shook his head good humouredly.

"Great Scott!" cried the athlete. "Why, I was first reserve for England against Wales, and I've *skippered* the 'Varsity all this year. But that's nothing! I didn't think there was a soul in England who didn't know Godfrey Staunton, the crack three-quarter, Cambridge, Blackheath, and five Internationals. Good Lord! Mr. Holmes, where HAVE you lived?"

Holmes laughed at the young giant's naive astonishment.

"You live in a different world to me, Mr. Overton – a sweeter and healthier one. My *ramifications* stretch out into many sections of society, but never, I am happy to say, into amateur sport, which is the best and soundest thing in England. However, your unexpected visit this morning shows me that even in that world of fresh air and *fair play,* there may be work for me to do. So now, my good sir, I beg you to sit down and to tell me, slowly and quietly, exactly what it is that has occurred, and how you desire that I should help you."

Young Overton's face assumed the bothered look of the man who is more accustomed to using his muscles than his wits, but by degrees, with many repetitions and *obscurities* which I may omit from his narrative, he laid his strange story before us.

"It's this way, Mr. Holmes. As I have said, I am the skip-per of the Rugger team of Cambridge 'Varsity, and Godfrey Staunton is my best man. Tomorrow we play Oxford. Yesterday we all came up, and we settled at Bentley's pri-vate hotel. At ten o'clock, I went around and saw that all the fellows had gone to roost, for I believe in strict training and plenty of sleep to keep a team fit. I had a word or two with Godfrey before he turned in. He seemed to me to be pale and bothered. I asked him what was the matter. He said he was all right – just a touch of headache. I bade him good-night and left him. Half an hour later, the porter tells me that a rough-looking man with a beard called with a note for Godfrey. He had not gone to bed, and the note was taken to his room. Godfrey read it, and fell back in a chair as if he had been *pole-axed.* The porter was so scared that he was going to fetch me, but Godfrey stopped him, had a drink of water, and pulled himself together. Then he went downstairs, said a few words to the man who was waiting in the hall, and the two of them went off together. The last that the porter saw of them, they were almost running down the street in the direction of the

Obscurities - *Uncertainties*
Roost - *A large cage*
Pole - axed - Moved *with a shafted weapon*
Skippered – *Captained*
Ramifications – *Consequences*

Strand. This morning Godfrey's room was empty, his bed had never been slept in, and his things were all just as I had seen them the night before.

He had gone off at a moment's notice with this stranger, and no word has come from him since. I don't believe he will ever come back. He was a sportsman, was Godfrey, down to his marrow, and he wouldn't have stopped his training and let in his skipper if it were not for some cause that was too strong for him. No: I feel as if he were gone for good, and we should never see him again."

Sherlock Holmes listened with the deepest attention to this singular narrative.

"What did you do?" he asked.

"I wired to Cambridge to learn if anything had been heard of him there. I have had an answer. No one has seen him."

"Could he have got back to Cambridge?"

"Yes, there is a late train – quarter-past eleven."

"But, so far as you can ascertain, he did not take it?"

"No, he has not been seen."

"What did you do next?"

"I wired to Lord Mount-James."

"Why to Lord Mount-James?"

"Godfrey is an orphan, and Lord Mount-James is his nearest relative – his uncle, I believe." "Indeed. This throws new light upon the matter. Lord Mount-James is one of the richest men in England."

"So I've heard Godfrey say."

"And your friend was closely related?"

"Yes, he was his heir, and the old boy is nearly eighty – *cram full* of *gout*, too. They say he could chalk his billiard-cue with his knuckles. He never allowed Godfrey a shilling in his life, for he is an absolute miser, but it will all come to him right enough."

"Have you heard from Lord Mount-James?"

"No." "What motive could your friend have in going to Lord Mount-James?"

"Well, something was worrying him the night before, and if it was to do with money it is possible that he would make for his

Cram full –
Completely full
Gout – *A medical condition causing swelling and pain in the joints*

nearest relative, who had so much of it, though from all I have heard he would not have much chance of getting it. Godfrey was not fond of the old man. He would not go if he could help it."

"Well, we can soon determine that. If your friend was going to his relative, Lord Mount-James, you have then to explain the visit of this rough-looking fellow at so late an hour, and the agitation that was caused by his coming."

Cyril Overton pressed his hands to his head. "I can make nothing of it," said he.

"Well, well, I have a clear day, and I shall be happy to look into the matter," said Holmes. "I should strongly recommend you to make your preparations for your match without reference to this young gentleman. It must, as you say, have been an *overpowering* necessity which tore him away in such a fashion, and the same necessity is likely to hold him away. Let us step round together to the hotel, and see if the porter can throw any fresh light upon the matter."

Sherlock Holmes was a past-master in the art of putting a humble witness at his ease, and very soon, in the privacy of Godfrey Staunton's abandoned room, he had extracted all that the porter had to tell. The visitor of the night before was not a gentleman, neither was he a workingman.

He was simply what the porter described as a "medium-looking chap," a man of fifty, beard *grizzled*, pale face, quietly dressed. He seemed himself to be agitated. The porter had observed his hand trembling when he had held out the note. Godfrey Staunton had *crammed* the note into his pocket. Staunton had not shaken hands with the man in the hall.

They had exchanged a few sentences, of which the porter had only distinguished the one word, "time." Then they had hurried off in the manner described. It was just half-past ten by the hall clock.

"Let me see," said Holmes, seating himself on Staunton's bed. "You are the day porter, are you not?"

"Yes, sir, I go off duty at eleven."

"The night porter saw nothing, I suppose?"

"No, sir, one theatre party came in late. No one else."

"Were you on duty all day yesterday?"

"Yes, sir."

Crammed - *To fill by force*
Overpowering – *Intense*
Grizzled – *Greyish*

"Did you take any messages to Mr. Staunton?"

"Yes, sir, one telegram."

"Ah! that's interesting. What o'clock was this?"

"About six."

"Where was Mr. Staunton when he received it?"

"Here in his room."

"Were you present when he opened it?"

"Yes, sir, I waited to see if there was an answer."

"Well, was there?"

"Yes, sir, he wrote an answer."

"Did you take it?"

"No, he took it himself."

"But he wrote it in your presence."

"Yes, sir. I was standing by the door, and he with his back turned at that table. When he had written it, he said: 'All right, porter, I will take this myself.'"

"What did he write it with?"

"A pen, sir."

"Was the telegraphic form one of these on the table?"

"Yes, sir, it was the top one."

Holmes rose. Taking the forms, he carried them over to the window and carefully examined that which was uppermost.

"It is a pity he did not write in pencil," said he, throwing them down again with a shrug of disappointment. "As you have no doubt frequently observed, Watson, the impression usually goes through – a fact which has **dissolved** many a happy marriage.

However, I can find no trace here. I rejoice, however, to perceive that he wrote with a broad-pointed quill pen, and I can hardly doubt that we will find some impression upon this blotting-pad. Ah, yes, surely this is the very thing!"

He tore off a strip of the blotting-paper and turned towards us the following *hieroglyphic*:

GRAPHIC

Dissolved – *Broke up*
Hieroglyphic –
Symbol or pictograph

Cyril Overton was much excited. "Hold it to the glass!" he cried.

"That is unnecessary," said Holmes. "The paper is thin, and the reverse will give the message. Here it is." He turned it over, and we read:

GRAPHIC [Stand by us for Gods sake]

"So that is the tail end of the telegram which Godfrey Staunton dispatched within a few hours of his disappearance. There are at least six words of the message which have escaped us; but what remains – 'Stand by us for God's sake!' – proves that this young man saw a formidable danger which approached him, and from which someone else could protect him. 'US,' mark you! Another person was involved.

Who should it be but the pale-faced, bearded man, who seemed himself in so nervous a state? What, then, is the connection between Godfrey Staunton and the bearded man? And what is the third source from which each of them sought for help against pressing danger? Our inquiry has already narrowed down to that."

"We have only to find to whom that telegram is addressed," I suggested.

"Exactly, my dear Watson. Your reflection, though profound, had already crossed my mind. But I daresay, it may have come to your notice that, *counterfoil* of another man's message, there may be some disinclination on the part of the officials to oblige you. There is so much red tape in these matters. However, I have no doubt that with a little delicacy and finesse, the end may be attained. Meanwhile, I should like in your presence, Mr. Overton, to go through these papers which have been left upon the table."

There were a number of letters, bills, and notebooks, which Holmes turned over and examined with quick, nervous fingers and darting, penetrating eyes. "Nothing here," he said, at last. "By the way, I suppose your friend was a healthy young fellow – nothing *amiss* with him?"

"Sound as a bell."

"Have you ever known him ill?"

"Not a day. He has been laid up with a hack, and once he slipped his knee-cap, but that was nothing."

Parson - *A member of the clergy*
Amiss - *Out of the right/proper course*
Twitching - *A quick, short movement*
Counterfoil – *The part of a cheque, etc. that is retained by the issuer*
Querulous – *Difficult*

"Perhaps, he was not so strong as you suppose. I should think he may have had some secret trouble. With your assent, I will put one or two of these papers in my pocket, in case they should bear upon our future inquiry."

"One moment – one moment!" cried a *querulous* voice, and we looked up to find a queer little old man, jerking and *twitching* in the doorway. He was dressed in rusty black, with a very broad-brimmed top-hat and a loose white necktie – the whole effect being that of a very rustic *parson* or of an undertaker's mute. Yet, in spite of his shabby and even absurd appearance, his voice had a sharp **crackle**, and his manner a quick intensity which commanded attention.

"Who are you, sir, and by what right do you touch this gentleman's papers?" he asked.

"I am a private detective, and I am endeavouring to explain his disappearance."

"Oh, you are, are you? And who instructed you, eh?"

"This gentleman, Mr. Staunton's friend, was referred to me by Scotland Yard."

"Who are you, sir?"

"I am Cyril Overton."

"Then it is you who sent me a telegram. My name is Lord Mount-James. I came around as quickly as the Bayswater bus would bring me. So you have instructed a detective?"

"Yes, sir."

"And are you prepared to meet the cost?"

"I have no doubt, sir, that my friend, Godfrey, when we find him, will be prepared to do that." "But if he is never found, eh? Answer me that!"

"In that case, no doubt his family –"

"Nothing of the sort, sir!" screamed the little man. "Don't look to me for a penny – not a penny! You understand that, Mr. Detective! I am all the family that this young man has got, and I tell you that I am not responsible. If he has any expectations, it is due to the fact that I have never wasted money, and I do not propose to begin to do so now. As to those papers with which you are *making so free*, I may tell you that in case there should be anything of any value among them, you will be held strictly to account for what you do with them."

Crackle – *To make a succession of sharp snapping noises*
Making so free – *Using without control*

Greatest   Adventure   Stories   of   Sherloc

"Very good, sir," said Sherlock Holmes. "May I ask, in the meanwhile, whether you have yourself any theory to account for this young man's disappearance?"

"No, sir, I have not. He is big enough and old enough to look after himself, and if he is so foolish as to lose himself, I entirely refuse to accept the responsibility of hunting for him."

"I quite understand your position," said Holmes, with a mischievous twinkle in his eyes. "Perhaps, you don't quite understand mine. Godfrey Staunton appears to have been a poor man. If he has been kidnapped, it could not have been for anything which he himself possesses. The fame of your wealth has gone abroad, Lord Mount-James, and it is entirely possible that a gang of thieves have secured your nephew in order to gain from him some information as to your house, your habits, and your treasure."

The face of our unpleasant little visitor turned as white as his neckcloth.

"Heavens, sir, what an idea! I never thought of such villainy! What inhuman rogues there are in the world! But Godfrey is a fine lad – a staunch lad. Nothing would induce him to give his old uncle away. I'll have the plate moved over to the bank this evening. In the meantime, spare no pains, Mr. Detective! I beg you to leave no stone unturned to bring him safely back. As to money, well, so far as a *fiver* or even a *tenner* goes you can always look to me."

Even in his *chastened* frame of mind, the noble miser could give us no information which could help us, for he knew little of the private life of his nephew. Our only clue lay in the *truncated* telegram, and with a copy of this in his hand, Holmes set forth to find a second link for his chain. We had shaken off Lord Mount-James, and Overton had gone to consult with the other members of his team over the misfortune which had befallen them.

There was a telegraph-office at a short distance from the hotel. We halted outside it.

"It's worth trying, Watson," said Holmes. "Of course, with a warrant, we could demand to see the counterfoils, but we have not reached that stage yet. I don't suppose they remember faces in so busy a place. Let us venture it."

Tenner - *A 10 - dollar bill or a 10 - pound note*
Fiver - *A 5 - pound note*
Grating - *A fixed frame of bars*
Sheaf - *A bundle/ cluster*
Chastened – *Punished*
Truncated – *Shortened*

"I am sorry to trouble you," said he, in his blandest manner, to the young woman behind the **grating**; "there is some small mistake about a telegram I sent yesterday. I have had no answer, and I very much fear that I must have omitted to put my name at the end. Could you tell me if this was so?"

The young woman turned over a **sheaf** of counterfoils.

"What o'clock was it?" she asked.

"A little after six."

"Whom was it to?"

Holmes put his finger to his lips and glanced at me. "The last words in it were 'For God's sake'," he whispered, confidentially; "I am very anxious at getting no answer."

The young woman separated one of the forms.

"This is it. There is no name," said she, smoothing it out upon the counter.

"Then that, of course, accounts for my getting no answer," said Holmes. "Dear me, how very stupid of me, to be sure! Good-morning, miss, and many thanks for having relieved my mind." He **chuckled** and rubbed his hands when we found ourselves in the street once more. "Well?" I asked.

"We progress, my dear Watson, we progress. I had seven different schemes for getting a glimpse of that telegram, but I could hardly hope to succeed the very first time."

"And what have you gained?"

"A starting-point for our investigation." He hailed a cab. "King's Cross Station," said he.

"We have a journey, then?"

"Yes, I think we must run down to Cambridge together. All the indications seem to me to point in that direction."

"Tell me," I asked, as we **rattled** up Gray's Inn Road, "have you any suspicion yet as to the cause of the disappearance? I don't think that among all our cases, I have known one where the motives are more obscure. Surely, you don't really imagine that he may be kidnapped in order to give information against his wealthy uncle?"

"I confess, my dear Watson, that that does not appeal to me as a very probable explanation. It struck me, however, as being the one which was most likely to interest that exceedingly unpleasant old person."

Chuckled - *To laugh softly*
Concocted - *To devise, make up*
Ruffians - *A tough, lawless person*
Ransom - *The sum price paid or demanded*
Rattled – *Upset*
Betting – *Gambling*

Greatest   Adventure   Stories   of   Sherloc

"It certainly did that; but what are your alternatives?"

"I could mention several. You must admit that it is curious and suggestive that this incident should occur on the eve of this important match, and should involve the only man whose presence seems essential to the success of the side. It may, of course, be a coincidence, but it is interesting.

Amateur sport is free from **betting**, but a good deal of outside betting goes on among the public, and it is possible that it might be worth someone's while to get at a player as the ruffians of the turf get at a race-horse. There is one explanation. A second very obvious one is that this young man really is the heir of a great property, however modest his means may at present be, and it is not impossible that a plot to hold him for ransom might be **concocted**."

"These theories take no account of the telegram."

"Quite true, Watson. The telegram still remains the only solid thing with which we have to deal, and we must not permit our attention to wander away from it. It is to gain light upon the purpose of this telegram that we are now upon our way to Cambridge. The path of our investigation is at present obscure, but I shall be very much surprised if before evening we have not cleared it up, or made a considerable advance along it."

It was already dark when we reached the old university city. Holmes took a cab at the station and ordered the man to drive to the house of Dr. Leslie Armstrong. A few minutes later, we had stopped at a large mansion in the busiest **thoroughfare**. We were shown in, and after a long wait were at last admitted into the consulting-room, where we found the doctor seated behind his table.

It argues the degree in which I had lost touch with my profession that the name of Leslie Armstrong was unknown to me. Now I am aware that he is not only one of the heads of the medical school of the university, but a thinker of European reputation in more than one branch of science.

Yet even without knowing his brilliant record, one could not fail to be impressed by a mere glance at the man, the square, massive face, the brooding eyes under the thatched brows, and the granite moulding of the inflexible jaw. A man of deep character, a man with an alert mind, grim, ascetic,

Thoroughfare –
Main road, Highway
Formidable –
Strong, Powerful

self-contained, *formidable* – so I read Dr. Leslie Armstrong. He held my friend's card in his hand, and he looked up with no very pleased expression upon his *dour* features.

"I have heard your name, Mr. Sherlock Holmes, and I am aware of your profession – one of which I by no means approve."

"In that, Doctor, you will find yourself in agreement with every criminal in the country," said my friend, quietly.

"So far as your efforts are directed towards the suppression of crime, sir, they must have the support of every reasonable member of the community, though I cannot doubt that the official machinery is amply sufficient for the purpose. Where your calling is more open to criticism is when you *pry* into the secrets of private individuals, when you *rake* up family matters which are better hidden, and when you incidentally waste the time of men who are more busy than yourself. At the present moment, for example, I should be writing a *treatise* instead of conversing with you."

"No doubt, Doctor; and yet the conversation may prove more important than the treatise. Incidentally, I may tell you that we are doing the reverse of what you very justly blame, and that we are endeavouring to prevent anything like public exposure of private matters which must necessarily follow when once the case is fairly in the hands of the official police. You may look upon me simply as an irregular pioneer, who goes in front of the regular forces of the country. I have come to ask you about Mr. Godfrey Staunton."

"What about him?"

"You know him, do you not?"

"He is an intimate friend of mine."

"You are aware that he has disappeared?"

"Ah, indeed!" There was no change of expression in the *rugged* features of the doctor.

"He left his hotel last night – he has not been heard of."

"No doubt he will return."

"Tomorrow is the 'Varsity football match."

"I have no sympathy with these childish games. The young man's fate interests me deeply, since I know him and like him. The football match does not come within my horizon at all."

Treatise – *Thesis*
Rugged – *Uneven*

"I claim your sympathy, then, in my investigation of Mr. Staunton's fate. Do you know where he is?"

"Certainly not."

"You have not seen him since yesterday?"

"No, I have not."

"Was Mr. Staunton a healthy man?"

"Absolutely." "Did you ever know him ill?"

"Never."

Holmes popped a sheet of paper before the doctor's eyes. "Then perhaps you will explain this receipted bill for thirteen guineas, paid by Mr. Godfrey Staunton last month to Dr. Leslie Armstrong, of Cambridge. I picked it out from among the papers upon his desk."

The doctor flushed with anger.

"I do not feel that there is any reason why I should render an explanation to you, Mr. Holmes."

Holmes replaced the bill in his notebook. "If you prefer a public explanation, it must come sooner or later," said he. "I have already told you that I can *hush up* that which others will be bound to publish, and you would really be wiser to take me into your complete confidence."

"I know nothing about it."

"Did you hear from Mr. Staunton in London?"

"Certainly not."

"Dear me, dear me – the post office again!" Holmes sighed, wearily. "A most urgent telegram was dispatched to you from London by Godfrey Staunton at six-fifteen yesterday evening – a telegram which is undoubtedly associated with his disappearance and yet you have not had it. It is most *culpable*. I shall certainly go down to the office here and register a complaint."

Dr. Leslie Armstrong sprang up from behind his desk, and his dark face was crimson with fury.

"I'll trouble you to walk out of my house, sir," said he. "You can tell your employer, Lord Mount-James, that I do not wish to have anything to do either with him or with his agents. No, sir – not another word!" He rang the bell furiously. "John, show these gentlemen out!" A *pompous* butler ushered

Dejected - *Sad or depressed*
Hush up - *Suppress*
Exhausted - *Tired*
Culpable – *Guilty*
Pompous – *Arrogant*

us severely to the door, and we found ourselves in the street. Holmes burst out laughing.

"Dr. Leslie Armstrong is certainly a man of energy and character," said he. "I have not seen a man who, if he turns his talents that way, was more calculated to fill the gap left by the illustrious Moriarty. And now, my poor Watson, here we are, stranded and friendless in this inhospitable town, which we cannot leave without abandoning our case. This little inn just opposite Armstrong's house is singularly adapted to our needs. If you would engage a front room and purchase the necessaries for the night, I may have time to make a few inquiries."

These few inquiries proved, however, to be a more lengthy proceeding than Holmes had imagined, for he did not return to the inn until nearly nine o'clock. He was pale and *dejected*, stained with dust, and *exhausted* with hunger and fatigue. A cold supper was ready upon the table, and when his needs were satisfied and his pipe alight, he was ready to take that half comic and wholly philosophic view which was natural to him when his affairs were going *awry*. The sound of carriage wheels caused him to rise and glance out of the window. A *brougham* and pair of grays, under the glare of a gas-lamp, stood before the doctor's door.

"It's been out three hours," said Holmes; "started at half-past six, and here it is back again. That gives a radius of ten or twelve miles, and he does it once, or sometimes twice, a day."

"No unusual thing for a doctor in practice."

"But Armstrong is not really a doctor in practice. He is a lecturer and a consultant, but he does not care for general practice, which distracts him from his literary work. Why, then, does he make these long journeys, which must be exceedingly *irksome* to him, and who is it that he visits?"

"His coachman –"

"My dear Watson, can you doubt that it was to him that I first applied? I do not know whether it came from his own innate *depravity* or from the promptings of his master, but he was rude enough to set a dog at me. Neither dog nor man liked the look of my stick, however, and the matter fell through. Relations were strained after that, and further inquiries out of the question.

Scintillating - *Sparkling or shining*
Discreet - *Careful*
Sardonic - *Cynical, Sarcastic*
Irksome - *Irritating*
Mortifying - *Embarrassing*
Depravity - *Morally corrupt act*
Awry – *Gone off track*
Brougham – *A horse-drawn carriage*

Greatest Adventure Stories of Sherloc

All that I have learned I got from a friendly native in the yard of our own inn. It was he who told me of the doctor's habits and of his daily journey. At that instant, to give point to his words, the carriage came round to the door."

"Could you not follow it?"

"Excellent, Watson! You are **scintillating** this evening. The idea did cross my mind. There is, as you may have observed, a bicycle shop next to our inn. Into this I rushed, engaged a bicycle, and was able to get started before the carriage was quite out of sight.

I rapidly overtook it, and then, keeping at a **discreet** distance of a hundred yards or so, I followed its lights until we were clear of the town. We had got well out on the country road, when a somewhat **mortifying** incident occurred.

The carriage stopped, the doctor alighted, walked swiftly back to where I had also halted, and told me in an excellent **sardonic** fashion that he feared the road was narrow, and that he hoped his carriage did not impede the passage of my bicycle. Nothing could have been more admirable than his way of putting it. I at once rode past the carriage, and, keeping to the main road, I went on for a few miles, and then halted in a convenient place to see if the carriage passed.

There was no sign of it, however, and so it became evident that it had turned down one of several side roads which I had observed. I rode back, but again saw nothing of the carriage, and now, as you perceive, it has returned after me. Of course, I had at the outset no particular reason to connect these journeys with the disappearance of Godfrey Staunton, and was only inclined to investigate them on the general grounds that everything which concerns Dr. Armstrong is at present of interest to us, but, now that I find he keeps so keen a look-out upon anyone who may follow him on these **excursions**, the affair appears more important, and I shall not be satisfied until I have made the matter clear."

"We can follow him tomorrow."

"Can we? It is not so easy as you seem to think. You are not familiar with Cambridgeshire scenery, are you? It does not lend itself to concealment. All this country that I passed over to-night is as flat and clean as the palm of your hand, and the

Excursions – *Expeditions*
Dogging – *Following somebody*

man we are following is no fool, as he very clearly showed *to-night.*

I have wired to Overton to let us know any fresh London developments at this address, and in the meantime, we can only concentrate our attention upon Dr. Armstrong, whose name the obliging young lady at the office allowed me to read upon the counterfoil of Staunton's urgent message.

He knows where the young man is – to that I'll swear, and if he knows, then it must be our own fault if we cannot manage to know also. At present, it must be admitted that the odd trick is in his possession, and, as you are aware, Watson, it is not my habit to leave the game in that condition."

And yet the next day brought us no nearer to the solution of the mystery. A note was handed in after breakfast, which Holmes passed across to me with a smile.

SIR [it ran]:

I can assure you that you are wasting your time in *dogging* my movements. I have, as you discovered last night, a window at the back of my brougham, and if you desire a twenty-mile ride which will lead you to the spot from which you started, you have only to follow me.

Meanwhile, I can inform you that no spying upon me can in any way help Mr. Godfrey Staunton, and I am convinced that the best service you can do to that gentleman is to return at once to London and to report to your employer that you are unable to trace him. Your time in Cambridge will certainly be wasted.

Yours faithfully,
LESLIE ARMSTRONG.

"An outspoken, honest *antagonist* is the doctor," said Holmes. "Well, well, he excites my curiosity, and I must really know before I leave him."

"His carriage is at his door now," said I. "There he is stepping into it. I saw him glance up at our window as he did so. Suppose I try my luck upon the bicycle?"

"No, no, my dear Watson! With all respect for your natural *acumen*, I do not think that you are quite a match for the worthy doctor. I think that possibly I can attain our end by

Antagonist – *Enemy*
Acumen – *Insight*

some independent explorations of my own. I am afraid that I must leave you to your own devices, as the appearance of TWO inquiring strangers upon a sleepy countryside might excite more gossip than I care for.

No doubt you will find some sights to amuse you in this *venerable* city, and I hope to bring back a more favourable report to you before evening." Once more, however, my friend was destined to be disappointed. He came back at night weary and unsuccessful.

"I have had a blank day, Watson. Having got the doctor's general direction, I spent the day in visiting all the villages upon that side of Cambridge, and comparing notes with publicans and other local news agencies. I have covered some ground. Chesterton, Histon, Waterbeach, and Oakington have each been explored, and have each proved disappointing. The daily appearance of a brougham and pair could hardly have been overlooked in such Sleepy Hollows. The doctor has scored once more. Is there a telegram for me?"

"Yes, I opened it. Here it is:

"Ask for Pompey from Jeremy Dixon, Trinity College.

"I don't understand it."

"Oh, it is clear enough. It is from our friend Overton, and is in answer to a question from me. I'll just send around a note to Mr. Jeremy Dixon, and then I have no doubt that our luck will turn. By the way, is there any news of the match?"

"Yes, the local evening paper has an excellent account in its last edition. Oxford won by a goal and two tries. The last sentences of the description say:

"The defeat of the Light Blues may be entirely attributed to the unfortunate absence of the crack International, Godfrey Staunton, whose want was felt at every instant of the game. The lack of combination in the three-quarter line and their weakness both in attack and defence more than *neutralized* the efforts of a heavy and hard-working pack."

"Then our friend Overton's *forebodings* have been justified," said Holmes. "Personally, I am in agreement with Dr. Armstrong, and football does not come within my horizon. Early to bed *to-night*, Watson, for I foresee that tomorrow may be an eventful day."

Leash - *A strap or cord*
Beagle - *A breed of small hound*
Forebodings - *fearful apprehensions*
Scouting - *The action of gathering information*
Squat - *Crouch, sit*
Neutralised – *Reduced the effect*
Hypodermic – *Beneath the skin*

I was horrified by my first glimpse of Holmes next morning, for he sat by the fire holding his tiny *hypodermic* syringe. I associated that instrument with the single weakness of his nature, and I feared the worst when I saw it glittering in his hand. He laughed at my expression of dismay and laid it upon the table.

"No, no, my dear fellow, there is no cause for alarm. It is not upon this occasion the instrument of evil, but it will rather prove to be the key which will unlock our mystery. On this syringe, I base all my hopes. I have just returned from a small scouting expedition, and everything is favourable. Eat a good breakfast, Watson, for I propose to get upon Dr. Armstrong's trail today, and once on it, I will not stop for rest or food until I run him to his burrow."

"In that case," said I, "we had best carry our breakfast with us, for he is making an early start. His carriage is at the door."

"Never mind. Let him go. He will be clever if he can drive where I cannot follow him. When you have finished, come downstairs with me, and I will introduce you to a detective who is a very eminent specialist in the work that lies before us."

When we descended, I followed Holmes into the stable yard, where he opened the door of a loose-box and led out a *squat*, lop-eared, white-and-tan dog, something between a beagle and a foxhound.

"Let me introduce you to Pompey," said he. "Pompey is the pride of the local draghounds – no very great flier, as his build will show, but a staunch hound on a scent. Well, Pompey, you may not be fast, but I expect you will be too fast for a couple of middle-aged London gentlemen, so I will take the liberty of fastening this leather *leash* to your collar.

Now, boy, come along, and show what you can do." He led him across to the doctor's door. The dog sniffed around for an instant, and then with a shrill whine of excitement started off down the street, *tugging* at his leash in his efforts to go faster. In half an hour, we were clear of the town and hastening down a country road.

"What have you done, Holmes?" I asked.

Threadbare – *(here)*
Thin and obvious
Venerable –
Admired

"A *threadbare* and *venerable* device, but useful upon occasion. I walked into the doctor's yard this morning, and shot my syringe full of aniseed over the hind wheel. A draghound will follow aniseed from here to John o'Groat's, and our friend, Armstrong, would have to drive through the Cam before he would shake Pompey off his trail. Oh, the cunning rascal! This is how he gave me the slip the other night."

The dog had suddenly turned out of the main road into a grass-grown lane. Half a mile farther this opened into another broad road, and the trail turned hard to the right in the direction of the town, which we had just quitted. The road took a sweep to the south of the town, and continued in the opposite direction to that in which we started.

"This **detour** has been entirely for our benefit, then?" said Holmes. "No wonder that my inquiries among those villagers led to nothing. The doctor has certainly played the game for all it is worth, and one would like to know the reason for such elaborate **deception**. This should be the village of Trumpington to the right of us. And, by Jove! here is the brougham coming around the corner. Quick, Watson – quick, or we are done!"

He sprang through a gate into a field, dragging the reluctant Pompey after him. We had hardly got under the shelter of the hedge when the carriage rattled past. I caught a glimpse of Dr. Armstrong within, his shoulders bowed, his head sunk on his hands, the very image of distress. I could tell by my companion's graver face that he also had seen.

"I fear there is some dark ending to our quest," said he. "It cannot be long before we know it. Come, Pompey! Ah, it is the cottage in the field!"

There could be no doubt that we had reached the end of our journey. Pompey ran about and whined eagerly outside the gate, where the marks of the brougham's wheels were still to be seen.

A footpath led across to the lonely cottage. Holmes tied the dog to the hedge, and we hastened onward. My friend knocked at the little rustic door, and knocked again without response. And yet the cottage was not deserted, for a low sound came to our ears – a kind of **drone** of misery and **despair** which was indescribably melancholy.

Holmes paused irresolute, and then he glanced back at the road which he had just traversed. A brougham was coming down it, and there could be no mistaking those gray horses.

Tangle - *Twisted together*
Despair - *Complete absence of hope*
Irresolue - *Uncertain*
Appalled - *Greatly dismayed*
Brawl - *Noisy fight or quarrel*
Drone – *Murmur*
Impunity – *Without any punishment*

"By Jove, the doctor is coming back!" cried Holmes. "That settles it. We are bound to see what it means before he comes."

He opened the door, and we stepped into the hall. The droning sound swelled louder upon our ears until it became one long, deep wail of distress. It came from upstairs. Holmes darted up, and I followed him. He pushed open a half-closed door, and we both stood *appalled* at the sight before us.

A woman, young and beautiful, was lying dead upon the bed. Her calm pale face, with dim, wide-opened blue eyes, looked upward from amid a great tangle of golden hair. At the foot of the bed, half sitting, half kneeling, his face buried in the clothes, was a young man, whose frame was racked by his sobs. So absorbed was he by his bitter grief, that he never looked up until Holmes's hand was on his shoulder.

"Are you Mr. Godfrey Staunton?"

"Yes, yes, I am – but you are too late. She is dead."

The man was so dazed that he could not be made to understand that we were anything but doctors who had been sent to his assistance. Holmes was endeavouring to utter a few words of consolation and to explain the alarm which had been caused to his friends by his sudden disappearance when there was a step upon the stairs, and there was the heavy, stern, questioning face of Dr. Armstrong at the door.

"So, gentlemen," said he, "you have attained your end and have certainly chosen a particularly delicate moment for your *intrusion*. I would not *brawl* in the presence of death, but I can assure you that if I were a younger man your monstrous conduct would not pass with *impunity*."

"Excuse me, Dr. Armstrong, I think we are a little at cross-purposes," said my friend, with dignity. "If you could step downstairs with us, we may each be able to give some light to the other upon this miserable affair."

A minute later, the grim doctor and ourselves were in the sitting room below.

"Well, sir?" said he.

"I wish you to understand, in the first place, that I am not employed by Lord Mount-James, and that my sympathies in this matter are entirely against that nobleman. When a man is

Breach - *Break, Pupture*
Consumption - *Utilisation*
Virulent - *Very poisonous*
Wrung – *Squeezed or twisted*
Compunction – *A feeling of remorse, guilt/regret*

lost it is my duty to ascertain his fate, but having done so, the matter ends so far as I am concerned, and so long as there is nothing criminal, I am much more anxious to hush up private scandals than to give them publicity.

If, as I imagine, there is no **breach** of the law in this matter, you can absolutely depend upon my discretion and my cooperation in keeping the facts out of the papers."

Dr. Armstrong took a quick step forward and *wrung* Holmes by the hand.

"You are a good fellow," said he. "I had misjudged you. I thank heaven that my *compunction* at leaving poor Staunton all alone in this plight caused me to turn my carriage back and so to make your acquaintance. Knowing as much as you do, the situation is very easily explained.

A year ago, Godfrey Staunton lodged in London for a time and became passionately attached to his landlady's daughter, whom he married. She was as good as she was beautiful and as intelligent as she was good. No man need be ashamed of such a wife. But Godfrey was the heir to this crabbed old nobleman, and it was quite certain that the news of his marriage would have been the end of his inheritance.

I knew the lad well, and I loved him for his many excellent qualities. I did all I could to help him to keep things straight. We did our very best to keep the thing from everyone, for, when once such a whisper gets about, it is not long before everyone has heard it. Thanks to this lonely cottage and his own discretion, Godfrey has up to now succeeded.

Their secret was known to no one save to me and to one excellent servant, who has at present gone for assistance to Trumpington. But at last, there came a terrible blow in the shape of dangerous illness to his wife. It was *consumption* of the most *virulent* kind. The poor boy was half crazed with grief, and yet he had to go to London to play this match, for he could not get out of it without explanations which would expose his secret. I tried to cheer him up by wire, and he sent me one in reply, imploring me to do all I could.

This was the telegram which you appear in some *inexplicable* way to have seen. I did not tell him how urgent the danger was, for I knew that he could do no good here, but

Frenzy - *Wild behaviour*
Grasped - *Hold firmly*
Inexplicable – *Mysterious*

I sent the truth to the girl's father, and he very *injudiciously* communicated it to Godfrey.

The result was that he came straight away in a state bordering on *frenzy*, and has remained in the same state, kneeling at the end of her bed, until this morning death put an end to her sufferings. That is all, Mr. Holmes, and I am sure that I can rely upon your discretion and that of your friend."

Holmes **grasped** the doctor's hand.

Injudiciously –
Unwisely

"Come, Watson," said he, and we passed from that house of grief into the pale sunlight of the winter day.

Food For Thought

If Holmes would not have visited Dr. Leslie Armstrong's yard and injected a syringe full of aniseeds over the hind wheel of the horse - driven coach, would he be able to solve the mystery of Godfrey Staunton's sudden disappearance?

An Understanding

Q. 1. Who was Cyril Overton? What made him to visit Holmes?

Ans. _____

_____

_____

_____

_____

Q. 2. Who was Godfrey Staunton? What happened to him?

Ans. _____

_____

_____

_____

_____

Q. 3. "No: I feel as if he were gone for good, and we should never see him again. Who said these words to whom? Who had 'gone for good' and what did the narrator of these lines fear about?

Ans. _____

_____

_____

_____

_____

Q. 4. Where did Dr. Leslie Armstrong go everyday once or sometimes, twice in his horse-driven coach? What happened when Watson and Holmes tried to follow him for the first time?

Ans. _____

_____

_____

_____

_____

The Adventure of the Engineer's Thumb

– Arthur Conan Doyle

OF all the problems which have been submitted to my friend, Mr. Sherlock Holmes, for solution during the years of our intimacy, there were only two which I was the means of introducing to his notice – that of Mr. Hatherley's thumb, and that of Colonel Warburton's madness. Of these the latter may have afforded a finer field for an acute and original observer, but the other was so strange in its *inception* and so dramatic in its details that it may be the more worthy of being placed upon record, even if it gave my friend fewer openings for those *deductive* methods of reasoning by which he achieved such remarkable results. The story has, I believe, been told more than once in the newspapers, but, like all such narratives, its effect is much less striking when set forth *en bloc* in a single half-column of print than when the facts slowly evolve before your own eyes, and the mystery clears gradually away as each new discovery furnishes a step which leads on to the complete truth. At the time the circumstances made a deep impression upon me, and the lapse of two years has hardly served to weaken the effect.

It was in the summer of '89, not long after my marriage, that the events occurred which I am now about to summarise. I had returned to civil practice and had finally abandoned Holmes in his Baker Street rooms, although I continually visited him and occasionally, even persuaded him to forgo his Bohemian habits so far as to come and visit us. My practice had steadily increased, and as I happened to live at no very great distance from Paddington Station, I got a few patients from among the officials. One of these, whom I had cured of a painful and lingering disease, was never weary of advertising my virtues and of endeavousring to send me on every sufferer over whom he might have any influence.

Deductive - *Based on*
Inception –
Beginning
En bloc – *All*
together

One morning, at a little before seven o'clock, I was awakened by the maid tapping at the door to announce that two men had come from Paddington and were waiting in the consulting-room. I dressed hurriedly, for I knew by experience that railway cases

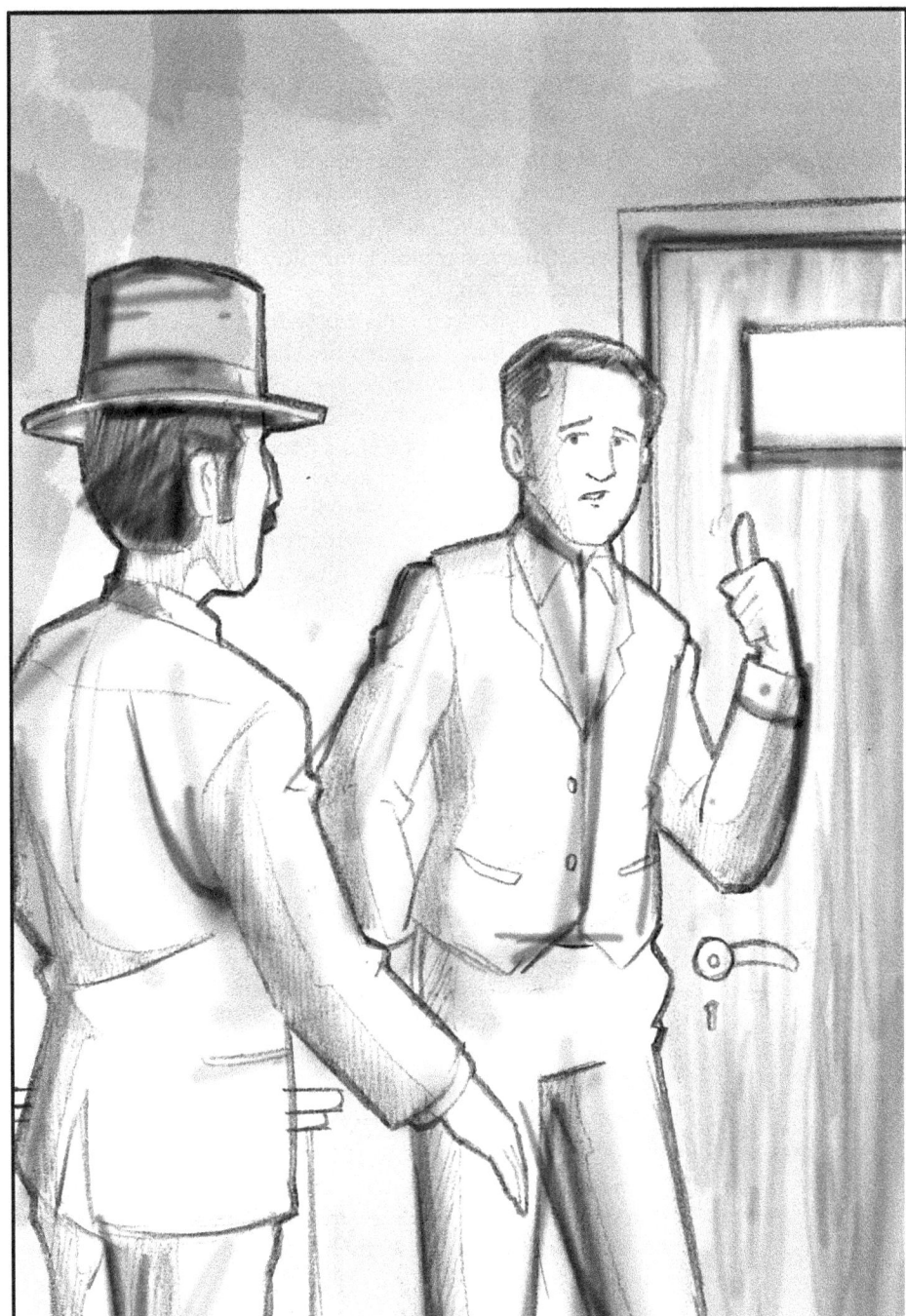

were seldom trivial, and hastened downstairs. As I *descended*, my old ally, the guard, came out of the room and closed the door tightly behind him.

"I've got him here," he whispered, jerking his thumb over his shoulder; "he's all right."

"What is it, then?" I asked, for his manner suggested that it was some strange creature which he had caged up in my room.

"It's a new patient," he whispered. "I thought I'd bring him round myself; then he couldn't slip away. There he is, all safe and sound. I must go now, Doctor; I have my dooties, just the same as you." And off he went, this trusty *tout*, without even giving me time to thank him. I entered my consulting-room and found a gentleman seated by the table. He was quietly dressed in a suit of *heather tweed* with a soft cloth cap which he had laid down upon my books. Around one of his hands he had a handkerchief wrapped, which was *mottled* all over with bloodstains. He was young, not more than five-and-twenty, I should say, with a strong, masculine face; but he was exceedingly pale and gave me the impression of a man who was suffering from some strong agitation, which it took all his strength of mind to control. "I am sorry to knock you up so early, Doctor," said he, "but I have had a very serious accident during the night. I came in by train this morning, and on inquiring at Paddington as to where I might find a doctor, a worthy fellow very kindly escorted me here. I gave the maid a card, but I see that she has left it upon the side-table."

I took it up and glanced at it. "Mr. Victor Hatherley, hydraulic engineer, 16A. Victoria Street (3d floor)." That was the name, style, and abode of my morning visitor. "I regret that I have kept you waiting," said I, sitting down in my library-chair. "You are fresh from a night journey, I understand, which is in itself a monotonous occupation."

"Oh, my night could not be called monotonous," said he, and laughed. He laughed very heartily, with a high, ringing note, leaning back in his chair and shaking his sides. All my medical instincts rose up against that laugh.

"Stop it!" I cried; "pull yourself together!" and I poured out some water from a *caraffe*.

It was useless, however. He was off in one of those hysterical outbursts which come upon a strong nature when some great crisis is over and gone. Presently he came to himself once more, very weary and pale-looking.

Heather tweed - *A coarse, rugged woollen fabric*
Tout – *One who publicizes something*
Caraffe – *A glass bottle*
Descended - *Move or fall downwards*
Mottled - *Marked with spots/smears*

Greatest   Adventure   Stories   of   Sherloc

"I have been making a fool of myself," he *gasped*.

"Not at all. Drink this." I dashed some brandy into the water, and the colour began to come back to his bloodless cheeks.

"That's better!" said he. "And now, Doctor, perhaps you would kindly attend to my thumb, or rather to the place where my thumb used to be."

He unwound the handkerchief and held out his hand. It gave even my hardened nerves a *shudder* to look at it. There were four protruding fingers and a horrid red, spongy surface where the thumb should have been. It had been *hacked* or torn right out from the roots.

"Good heavens!" I cried, "this is a terrible injury. It must have bled considerably."

"Yes, it did. I fainted when it was done, and I think that I must have been senseless for a long time. When I came to I found that it was still bleeding, so I tied one end of my handkerchief very tightly around the wrist and braced it up with a **twig**."

"Excellent! You should have been a surgeon."

"It is a question of hydraulics, you see, and came within my own province."

"This has been done," said I, examining the wound, "by a very heavy and sharp instrument."

"A thing like a *cleaver*," said he.

"An accident, I presume?"

"By no means."

"What! a murderous attack?"

"Very murderous indeed."

"You horrify me."

I sponged the wound, cleaned it, dressed it, and finally covered it over with cotton *wadding* and carbolized bandages. He lay back without *wincing*, though he bit his lip from time to time.

"How is that?" I asked when I had finished.

"Capital! Between your brandy and your bandage, I feel a new man. I was very weak, but I have had a good deal to go through."

"Perhaps you had better not speak of the matter. It is evidently trying to your nerves."

"Oh, no, not now. I shall have to tell my tale to the police; but, between ourselves, if it were not for the convincing evidence of this wound of mine, I should be surprised if they believed my

Hacked - *Cut with a heavy blow*

Shudder - *Tremble*

Gasped - *inhale suddenly*

Wadding - *Soft thick material used to line garments*

Wincing - *Shrink in pain*

Twig – *Branch*

Cleaver – *A heavy Knife*

statement, for it is a very extraordinary one, and I have not much in the way of proof with which to back it up; and, even if they believe me, the clues which I can give them are so vague that it is a question whether justice will be done."

"Ha!" cried I, "if it is anything in the nature of a problem which you desire to see solved, I should strongly recommend you to come to my friend, Mr. Sherlock Holmes, before you go to the official police."

"Oh, I have heard of that fellow," answered my visitor, "and I should be very glad if he would take the matter up, though of course, I must use the official police as well. Would you give me an introduction to him?"

"I'll do better. I'll take you around to him myself."

"I should be immensely obliged to you."

"We'll call a cab and go together. We shall just be in time to have a little breakfast with him. Do you feel equal to it?"

"Yes; I shall not feel easy until I have told my story."

"Then my servant will call a cab, and I shall be with you in an instant." I rushed upstairs, explained the matter shortly to my wife, and in five minutes, was inside a *hansom*, driving with my new acquaintance to Baker Street.

Sherlock Holmes was, as I expected, *lounging* about his sittingroom in his dressing-gown, reading the agony column of The Times and smoking his before-breakfast pipe, which was composed of all the *plugs* and *dottles* left from his smokes of the day before, all carefully dried and collected on the corner of the mantelpiece. He received us in his quietly genial fashion, ordered fresh *rashers* and eggs, and joined us in a hearty meal. When it was concluded, he settled our new acquaintance upon the sofa, placed a pillow beneath his head, and laid a glass of brandy and water within his reach.

"It is easy to see that your experience has been no common one, Mr. Hatherley," said he. "Pray, lie down there and make yourself absolutely at home. Tell us what you can, but stop when you are tired and keep up your strength with a little *stimulant*."

"Thank you," said my patient. "but I have felt another man since the doctor bandaged me, and I think that your breakfast has completed the cure. I shall take up as little of your valuable time as possible, so I shall start at once upon my peculiar experiences."

Holmes sat in his big armchair with the weary, heavy-lidded expression which **veiled** his keen and eager nature, while I sat

Stimulant – A drug that increases Physilogical activity
Hansom – A two-wheeled horse drawn carriage
Dottles – Tobacco ash

opposite to him, and we listened in silence to the strange story which our visitor detailed to us.

"You must know," said he, "that I am an orphan and a bachelor, residing alone in lodgings in London. By profession, I am a hydraulic engineer, and I have had considerable experience of my work during the seven years that I was apprenticed to Venner & Matheson, the well-known firm, of Greenwich. Two years ago, having served my time, and having also come into a fair sum of money through my poor father's death, I determined to start in business for myself and took professional chambers in Victoria Street.

"I suppose that everyone finds his first independent start in business a *dreary* experience. To me, it has been *exceptionally* so. During two years, I have had three consultations and one small job, and that is absolutely all that my profession has brought me. My gross takings amount to 27 pounds 10shillings. Every day, from nine in the morning until four in the afternoon, I waited in my little den, until at last my heart began to sink, and I came to believe that I should never have any practice at all.

"Yesterday, however, just as I was thinking of leaving the office, my clerk entered to say there was a gentleman waiting who wished to see me upon business. He brought up a card, too, with the name of 'Colonel Lysander Stark' engraved upon it. Close at his heels came the colonel himself, a man rather over the middle size, but of an exceeding thinness. I do not think that I have ever seen so thin a man. His whole face sharpened away into nose and chin, and the skin of his cheeks was drawn quite tense over his outstanding bones. Yet this *emaciation* seemed to be his natural habit, and due to no disease, for his eye was bright, his step brisk, and his bearing assured. He was plainly but neatly dressed, and his age, I should judge, would be nearer forty than thirty.

"'Mr. Hatherley?' said he, with something of a German accent. 'You have been recommended to me, Mr. Hatherley, as being a man who is not only *proficient* in his profession but is also discreet and capable of preserving a secret.'

"I bowed, feeling as flattered as any young man would at such an address. 'May I ask who it was who gave me so good a character?'

Ereary - *Depressing*
Exceptionally - *Exceedingly*
Veiled – *Covered or hidden*
Emaciation – *Extreme thinness*

"'Well, perhaps it is better that I should not tell you that just at this moment. I have it from the same source that you are both an orphan and a bachelor and are residing alone in London.'

"'That is quite correct,' I answered; 'but you will excuse me if I say that I cannot see how all this bears upon my professional qualifications. I understand that it was on a professional matter that you wished to speak to me?'

"'Undoubtedly so. But you will find that all I say is really to the point. I have a professional commission for you, but absolute secrecy is quite essential – absolute secrecy, you understand, and of course, we may expect that more from a man who is alone than from one who lives in the *bosom* of his family.'

"'If I promise to keep a secret,' said I, 'you may absolutely depend upon my doing so.'

"He looked very hard at me as I spoke, and it seemed to me that I had never seen so suspicious and questioning an eye.

"'Do you promise, then?' said he at last.

"'Yes, I promise.'

"'Absolute and complete silence before, during, and after? No reference to the matter at all, either in word or writing?'

"'I have already given you my word.'

"'Very good.' He suddenly sprang up, and darting like lightning across the room he flung open the door. The passage outside was empty.

"'That's all right,' said he, coming back. 'I know the clerks are sometimes curious as to their master's affairs. Now we can talk in safety.' He drew up his chair very close to mine and began to stare at me again with the same questioning and thoughtful look.

"A feeling of *repulsion*, and of something akin to fear had begun to rise within me at the strange *antics* of this fleshless man. Even my dread of losing a client could not restrain me from showing my impatience.

"'I beg that you will state your business, sir,' said I; 'my time is of value.' Heaven forgive me for that last sentence, but the words came to my lips.

"'How would fifty guineas for a night's work suit you?' he asked.

"'Most admirably.'

"'I say a night's work, but an hour's would be nearer the mark. I simply want your opinion about a hydraulic stamping

Bosom - *Heart or chest*

Repulsion – *Disgust*

Antics – *Tricks*

machine which has got out of gear. If you show us what is wrong, we shall soon set it right ourselves. What do you think of such a commission as that?'

"'The work appears to be light and the pay *munificent*.'

"'Precisely so. We shall want you to come tonight by the last train.'

"'Where to?'

"'To Eyford, in Berkshire. It is a little place near the borders of Oxfordshire, and within seven miles of Reading. There is a train from Paddington which would bring you there at about 11:15.'

"'Very good.'

"'I shall come down in a carriage to meet you.'

"'There is a drive, then?'

"'Yes, our little place is quite out in the country. It is a good seven miles from Eyford Station.'

"'Then we can hardly get there before midnight. I suppose there would be no chance of a train back. I should be compelled to stop the night.'

"'Yes, we could easily give you a shake-down.'

"'That is very awkward. Could I not come at some more convenient hour?'

"'We have judged it best that you should come late. It is to *recompense* you for any inconvenience that we are paying to you, a young and unknown man, a fee which would buy an opinion from the very heads of your profession. Still, of course, if you would like to draw out of the business, there is plenty of time to do so.'

"I thought of the fifty guineas, and of how very useful they would be to me. 'Not at all,' said I, 'I shall be very happy to accommodate myself to your wishes. I should like, however, to understand a little more clearly what it is that you wish me to do.'

"'Quite so. It is very natural that the pledge of secrecy which we have exacted from you should have aroused your curiosity. I have no wish to commit you to anything without your having it all laid before you. I suppose that we are absolutely safe from *eavesdroppers*?'

"'Entirely.'

"'Then the matter stands thus. You are probably aware that fuller's-earth is a valuable product, and that it is only found in one or two places in England?'

Munificent –
Generous
Recompense –
Reward

"'I have heard so.'

"'Some little time ago, I bought a small place – a very small place – within ten miles of Reading. I was fortunate enough to discover that there was a deposit of fuller's-earth in one of my fields. On examining it, however, I found that this deposit was a comparatively small one, and that it formed a link between two very much larger ones upon the right and left – both of them, however, in the grounds of my **neighbors**. These good people were absolutely ignorant that their land contained that which was quite as valuable as a gold-mine. Naturally, it was to my interest to buy their land before they discovered its true value, but unfortunately, I had no capital by which I could do this. I took a few of my friends into the secret, however, and they suggested that we should quietly and secretly work our own little deposit and that in this way we should earn the money which would enable us to buy the neighbouring fields. This we have now been doing for some time, and in order to help us in our operations we **erected** a hydraulic press. This press, as I have already explained, has got out of order, and we wish your advice upon the subject. We guard our secret very jealously, however, and if it once became known that we had hydraulic engineers coming to our little house, it would soon arouse inquiry, and then, if the facts came out, it would be goodbye to any chance of getting these fields and carrying out our plans. That is why I have made you promise me that you will not tell a human being that you are going to Eyford tonight. I hope that I make it all plain?'

"'I quite follow you,' said I. 'The only point which I could not quite understand was what use you could make of a hydraulic press in **excavating** fuller's-earth, which, as I understand, is dug out like gravel from a pit.'

"'Ah!' said he carelessly, 'we have our own process. We compress the earth into bricks, so as to remove them without revealing what they are. But that is a mere detail. I have taken you fully into my confidence now, Mr. Hatherley, and I have shown you how I trust you.' He rose as he spoke. 'I shall expect you, then, at Eyford at 11:15.'

"'I shall certainly be there.'

"'And not a word to a soul.' He looked at me with a last long, questioning gaze, and then, pressing my hand in a cold, **dank grasp,** he hurried from the room.

Eavesdroppers
- *Secret listeners to conversations*
Erected – *Raised*
Excavating –
Digging out

"Well, when I came to think it all over in cool blood I was very much astonished, as you may both think, at this sudden commission which had been entrusted to me. On the one hand, of course, I was glad, for the fee was at least tenfold what I should have asked had I set a price upon my own services, and it was possible that this order might lead to other ones. On the other hand, the face and manner of my patron had made an unpleasant impression upon me, and I could not think that his explanation of the fuller's-earth was sufficient to explain the necessity for my coming at midnight, and his extreme anxiety, lest I should tell anyone of my *errand*. However, I threw all fears to the winds, ate a hearty supper, drove to Paddington, and started off, having obeyed to the letter the *injunction* as to holding my tongue.

"At Reading I had to change not only my carriage but my station. However, I was in time for the last train to Eyford, and I reached the little dim-lit station after eleven o'clock. I was the only passenger who got out there, and there was no one upon the platform save a single sleepy porter with a lantern. As I passed out through the wicket gate, however, I found my acquaintance of the morning waiting in the shadow upon the other side. Without a word, he grasped my arm and hurried me into a carriage, the door of which was standing open. He drew up the windows on either side, tapped on the wood-work, and away we went as fast as the horse could go."

"One horse?" interjected Holmes.

"Yes, only one."

"Did you observe the colour?"

"Yes, I saw it by the sidelights when I was stepping into the carriage. It was a chestnut."

"Tired-looking or fresh?"

"Oh, fresh and glossy."

"Thank you. I am sorry to have interrupted you. Pray continue your most interesting statement."

"Away we went then, and we drove for at least an hour. Colonel Lysander Stark had said that it was only seven miles, but I should think, from the rate that we seemed to go, and from the time that we took, that it must have been nearer twelve. He sat at my side in silence all the time, and I was aware, more than once when I glanced in his direction, that he was looking at me with great intensity. The country roads seem to be not very good in

Errand - *Work*
Dank – *Damp*
Injunction – *Order*

that part of the world, for we *lurched* and jolted terribly. I tried to look out of the windows to see something of where we were, but they were made of *frosted* glass, and I could make out nothing save the occasional bright blur of a passing light. Now and then, I hazarded some remark to break the monotony of the journey, but the colonel answered only in monosyllables, and the conversation soon *flagged*. At last, however, the bumping of the road was exchanged for the crisp smoothness of a gravel-drive, and the carriage came to a stand. Colonel Lysander Stark sprang out, and, as I followed after him, pulled me swiftly into a porch which gaped in front of us. We stepped, as it were, right out of the carriage and into the hall, so that I failed to catch the most fleeting glance of the front of the house. The instant that I had crossed the threshold, the door slammed heavily behind us, and I heard faintly the rattle of the wheels as the carriage drove away.

"It was pitch dark inside the house, and the colonel *fumbled* about looking for matches and muttering under his breath. Suddenly a door opened at the other end of the passage, and a long, golden bar of light shot out in our direction. It grew broader, and a woman appeared with a lamp in her hand, which she held above her head, pushing her face forward and peering at us. I could see that she was pretty, and from the *gloss* with which the light shone upon her dark dress I knew that it was a rich material. She spoke a few words in a foreign tongue in a tone as though asking a question, and when my companion answered in a *gruff* monosyllable, she gave such a start that the lamp nearly fell from her hand. Colonel Stark went up to her, whispered something in her ear, and then, pushing her back into the room from whence she had come, he walked towards me again with the lamp in his hand.

"'Perhaps, you will have the kindness to wait in this room for a few minutes,' said he, throwing open another door. It was a quiet, little, plainly furnished room, with a round table in the centre, on which several German books were scattered. Colonel Stark laid down the lamp on the top of a harmonium beside the door. 'I shall not keep you waiting an instant,' said he, and vanished into the darkness.

"I glanced at the books upon the table, and in spite of my ignorance of German, I could see that two of them were treatises on science, the others being volumes of poetry. Then I walked across to the window, hoping that I might catch some glimpse of the countryside, but an oak shutter, heavily barred, was folded across

Gloss - *Bright sheen*
Fumbled - *To touch or handle nervously*
Gruff - *Hoarse or harsh*
Lurched – *stumbled*
Flagged – *Faded away*

it. It was a wonderfully silent house. There was an old clock ticking loudly somewhere in the passage, but otherwise everything was deadly still. A vague feeling of uneasiness began to steal over me. Who were these German people, and what were they doing living in this strange, out-of-the-way place? And where was the place? I was ten miles or so from Eyford, that was all I knew, but whether north, south, east, or west, I had no idea. For that matter, Reading, and possibly other large towns, were within that radius, so the place might not be so *secluded*, after all. Yet it was quite certain, from the absolute stillness, that we were in the country. I paced up and down the room, humming a tune under my breath to keep up my spirits and feeling that I was thoroughly earning my fifty-guinea fee.

"Suddenly, without any preliminary sound in the midst of the utter stillness, the door of my room swung slowly open. The woman was standing in the *aperture*, the darkness of the hall behind her, the yellow light from my lamp beating upon her eager and beautiful face. I could see at a glance that she was sick with fear, and the sight sent a chill to my own heart. She held up one shaking finger to warn me to be silent, and she shot a few whispered words of broken English at me, her eyes glancing back, like those of a frightened horse, into the gloom behind her.

"'I would go,' said she, trying hard, as it seemed to me, to speak calmly; 'I would go. I should not stay here. There is no good for you to do.'

"'But, madam,' said I, 'I have not yet done what I came for. I cannot possibly leave until I have seen the machine.'

"'It is not worth your while to wait,' she went on. 'You can pass through the door; no one *hinders*.' And then, seeing that I smiled and shook my head, she suddenly threw aside her constraint and made a step forward, with her hands wrung together. 'For the love of Heaven!' she whispered, 'get away from here before it is too late!'

"But I am somewhat *headstrong* by nature, and the more ready to engage in an affair when there is some obstacle in the way. I thought of my fifty-guinea fee, of my wearisome journey, and of the unpleasant night which seemed to be before me. Was it all to go for nothing? Why should I *slink* away without having carried out my commission, and without the payment which was my due? This woman might, for all I knew, be a *monomaniac*. With a stout bearing, therefore, though her manner had shaken me more than I cared to confess, I still shook my head and

Aperture – *Hole*
Hinders – *Delays*

declared my intention of remaining where I was. She was about to renew her *entreaties* when a door slammed overhead, and the sound of several footsteps was heard upon the stairs. She listened for an instant, threw up her hands with a despairing gesture, and vanished as suddenly and as noiselessly as she had come.

"The newcomers were Colonel Lysander Stark and a short thick man with a *chinchilla* beard growing out of the *creases* of his double chin, who was introduced to me as Mr. Ferguson.

"'This is my secretary and manager,' said the colonel. 'By the way, I was under the impression that I left this door shut just now. I fear that you have felt the draught.'

"'On the contrary,' said I, 'I opened the door myself because I felt the room to be a little close.' "He shot one of his suspicious looks at me. 'Perhaps, we had better proceed to business, then,' said he. 'Mr. Ferguson and I will take you up to see the machine.'

"'I had better put my hat on, I suppose.'

"'Oh, no, it is in the house.'

"'What, you dig fuller's-earth in the house?'

"'No, no. This is only where we compress it. But never mind that. All we wish you to do is to examine the machine and to let us know what is wrong with it.'

"We went upstairs together, the colonel first with the lamp, the fat manager and I behind him. It was a *labyrinth* of an old house, with corridors, passages, narrow winding staircases, and little low doors, the *thresholds* of which were hollowed out by the generations who had crossed them. There were no carpets and no signs of any furniture above the ground floor, while the plaster was peeling off the walls, and the damp was breaking through in green, unhealthy *blotches*. I tried to put on as unconcerned an air as possible, but I had not forgotten the warnings of the lady, even though I disregarded them, and I kept a keen eye upon my two companions. Ferguson appeared to be a *morose* and silent man, but I could see from the little that he said that he was at least a fellow-countryman.

"Colonel Lysander Stark stopped at last before a low door, which he unlocked. Within was a small, square room, in which the three of us could hardly get at one time. Ferguson remained outside, and the colonel ushered me in.

"'We are now,' said he, 'actually within the hydraulic press, and it would be a particularly unpleasant thing for us if anyone

Threshold - *At the outset*
Labyrinth - *An elaborate structure*
Headstrong – *Determined*
Monomaniac – *One who is obsessed with an idea or object*

were to turn it on. The ceiling of this small chamber is really the end of the descending piston, and it comes down with the force of many tons upon this metal floor. There are small lateral columns of water outside which receive the force, and which transmit and multiply it in the manner which is familiar to you. The machine goes readily enough, but there is some stiffness in the working of it, and it has lost a little of its force. Perhaps, you will have the goodness to look it over and to show us how we can set it right.'

"I took the lamp from him, and I examined the machine very thoroughly. It was indeed a gigantic one, and capable of exercising enormous pressure. When I passed outside, however, and pressed down the levers which controlled it, I knew at once by the whishing sound that there was a slight leakage, which allowed a *regurgitation* of water through one of the side cylinders. An examination showed that one of the india-rubber bands which was around the head of a driving-rod had shrunk so as not quite to fill the socket along which it worked. This was clearly the cause of the loss of power, and I pointed it out to my companions, who followed my remarks very carefully and asked several practical questions as to how they should proceed to set it right. When I had made it clear to them, I returned to the main chamber of the machine and took a good look at it to satisfy my own curiosity. It was obvious at a glance that the story of the fuller's earth was the merest fabrication, for it would be absurd to suppose that so powerful an engine could be designed for so inadequate a purpose. The walls were of wood, but the floor consisted of a large iron trough, and when I came to examine it I could see a crust of metallic deposit all over it. I had stooped and was scraping at this to see exactly what it was when I heard a muttered exclamation in German and saw the *cadaverous* face of the colonel looking down at me.

"'What are you doing there?' he asked.

"I felt angry at having been tricked by so elaborate a story as that which he had told me. 'I was admiring your fuller's-earth,' said I; 'I think that I should be better able to advise you as to your machine if I knew what the exact purpose was for which it was used.'

"The instant that I uttered the words I regretted the rashness of my speech. His face set hard, and a *baleful* light sprang up in his grey eyes.

"'Very well,' said he, 'you shall know all about the machine.' He took a step backward, slammed the little door, and turned the

Morose – *Miserable, Gloomy*
Regurgitation – *To cause to surge back*

key in the lock. I rushed towards it and pulled at the handle, but it was quite secure, and did not give in the least to my kicks and shoves. 'Hello!' I yelled. 'Hello! Colonel! Let me out!'

"And then suddenly in the silence I heard a sound which sent my heart into my mouth. It was the clank of the levers and the swish of the leaking cylinder. He had set the engine at work. The lamp still stood upon the floor where I had placed it when examining the trough. By its light I saw that the black ceiling was coming down upon me, slowly, jerkily, but, as none knew better than myself, with a force which must within a minute grind me to a shapeless pulp. I threw myself, screaming, against the door, and dragged with my nails at the lock. I *implored* the colonel to let me out, but the *remorseless* clanking of the levers drowned my cries. The ceiling was only a foot or two above my head, and with my hand upraised I could feel its hard, rough surface. Then it flashed through my mind that the pain of my death would depend very much upon the position in which I met it. If I lay on my face the weight would come upon my spine, and I shuddered to think of that dreadful *snap*. Easier the other way, perhaps; and yet, had I the nerve to lie and look up at that deadly black shadow wavering down upon me? Already I was unable to stand erect, when my eye caught something which brought a gush of hope back to my heart.

"I have said that though the floor and ceiling were of iron, the walls were of wood. As I gave a last hurried glance around, I saw a thin line of yellow light between two of the boards, which broadened and broadened as a small panel was pushed backward. For an instant, I could hardly believe that here was indeed a door which led away from death. The next instant, I threw myself through, and lay half-fainting upon the other side. The panel had closed again behind me, but the crash of the lamp, and a few moments afterwards, the clang of the two slabs of metal, told me how narrow had been my escape.

"I was recalled to myself by a frantic plucking at my wrist, and I found myself lying upon the stone floor of a narrow corridor, while a woman bent over me and tugged at me with her left hand, while she held a candle in her right. It was the same good friend whose warning I had so foolishly rejected.

"'Come! come!' she cried breathlessly. 'They will be here in a moment. They will see that you are not there. Oh, do not waste the so-precious time, but come!'

Implored - *Begged*
Remorseless - *No pity or compassion*
Snap - *To make a brisk, sharp, cracking sound*
Cadaverous – *Ashen, ghostlike*
Baleful – *Threatening*

"This time, at least, I did not scorn her advice. I staggered to my feet and ran with her along the corridor and down a winding stair. The latter led to another broad passage, and just as we reached it, we heard the sound of running feet and the shouting of two voices, one answering the other from the floor on which we were and from the one beneath. My guide stopped and looked about her like one who is at her wit's end. Then she threw open a door which led into a bedroom, through the window of which the moon was shining brightly.

"'It is your only chance,' said she. 'It is high, but it may be that you can jump it.'

"As she spoke a light sprang into view at the further end of the passage, and I saw the lean figure of Colonel Lysander Stark rushing forward with a lantern in one hand and a weapon like a butcher's cleaver in the other. I rushed across the bedroom, flung open the window, and looked out. How quiet and sweet and wholesome the garden looked in the moonlight, and it could not be more than thirty feet down. I *clambered* out upon the *sill*, but I hesitated to jump until I should have heard what passed between my saviour and the *ruffian* who pursued me. If she were *ill-used*, then at any risks, I was determined to go back to her assistance. The thought had hardly flashed through my mind before he was at the door, pushing his way past her; but she threw her arms round him and tried to hold him back.

"'Fritz! Fritz!' she cried in English, 'remember your promise after the last time. You said it should not be again. He will be silent! Oh, he will be silent!'

"'You are mad, Elise!' he shouted, struggling to break away from her. 'You will be the ruin of us. He has seen too much. Let me pass, I say!' He *dashed* her to one side, and, rushing to the window, cut at me with his heavy weapon. I had let myself go, and was hanging by the hands to the sill, when his blow fell. I was conscious of a dull pain, my grip loosened, and I fell into the garden below.

"I was shaken but not hurt by the fall; so I picked myself up and rushed off among the bushes as hard as I could run, for I understood that I was far from being out of danger yet. Suddenly, however, as I ran, a deadly dizziness and sickness came over me. I glanced down at my hand, which was throbbing painfully, and then, for the first time, saw that my thumb had been cut off and that the blood was pouring from my wound. I endeavoured to tie my handkerchief around it, but there came a sudden buzzing

Sill - *The basis/ foundation*
Ruffian - *a tough or rowdy person*
Clambered – *Climbed*
Ill-used – *Mistreated or harmed*

in my ears, and the next moment I fell in a dead faint among the rose-bushes.

"How long I remained unconscious, I cannot tell. It must have been a very long time, for the moon had sunk, and a bright morning was breaking when I came to myself. My clothes were all *sodden* with dew, and my coat-sleeve was drenched with blood from my wounded thumb. The smarting of it recalled in an instant all the particulars of my night's adventure, and I sprang to my feet with the feeling that I might hardly yet be safe from my pursuers. But to my astonishment, when I came to look around me, neither house nor garden were to be seen. I had been lying in an angle of the hedge close by the highroad, and just a little lower down was a long building, which proved, upon my approaching it, to be the very station at which I had arrived upon the previous night. Were it not for the ugly wound upon my hand, all that had passed during those dreadful hours might have been an evil dream.

"Half dazed, I went into the station and asked about the morning train. There would be one to Reading in less than an hour. The same porter was on duty, I found, as had been there when I arrived. I inquired of him whether he had ever heard of Colonel Lysander Stark. The name was strange to him. Had he observed a carriage the night before waiting for me? No, he had not. Was there a police-station anywhere near? There was one about three miles off.

"It was too far for me to go, weak and ill as I was. I determined to wait until I got back to town before telling my story to the police. It was a little past six when I arrived, so I went first to have my wound dressed, and then the doctor was kind enough to bring me along here. I put the case into your hands and shall do exactly what you advise."

We both sat in silence for some little time after listening to this extraordinary narrative. Then Sherlock Holmes pulled down from the shelf one of the *ponderous* commonplace books in which he placed his cuttings.

"Here is an advertisement which will interest you," said he. "It appeared in all the papers about a year ago. Listen to this: 'Lost, on the 9th inst., Mr. Jeremiah Hayling, aged twenty-six, a hydraulic engineer. Left his lodgings at ten o'clock at night, and has not been heard of since. Was dressed in,' etc., etc. Ha! That

Dashed – *Rushed*
Sodden – *Wet*

represents the last time that the colonel needed to have his machine *overhauled*, I fancy."

"Good heavens!" cried my patient. "Then that explains what the girl said."

"Undoubtedly. It is quite clear that the colonel was a cool and desperate man, who was absolutely determined that nothing should stand in the way of his little game, like those out-and-out pirates, who will leave no survivor from a captured ship. Well, every moment now is precious, so if you feel equal to it we shall go down to Scotland Yard at once as a preliminary to starting for Eyford."

Some three hours or so afterwards we were all in the train together, bound from Reading to the little Berkshire village. There were Sherlock Holmes, the hydraulic engineer, Inspector Bradstreet, of Scotland Yard, a plain-clothes man, and myself. Bradstreet had spread an *ordnance* map of the county out upon the seat and was busy with his compasses drawing a circle with Eyford for its centre.

"There you are," said he. "That circle is drawn at a radius of ten miles from the village. The place we want must be somewhere near that line. You said ten miles, I think, sir."

"It was an hour's good drive."

"And you think that they brought you back all that way when you were unconscious?"

"They must have done so. I have a confused memory, too, of having been lifted and conveyed somewhere."

"What I cannot understand," said I, "is why they should have spared you when they found you lying fainting in the garden. Perhaps, the villain was softened by the woman's entreaties."

"I hardly think that likely. I never saw a more *inexorable* face in my life."

"Oh, we shall soon clear up all that," said Bradstreet. "Well, I have drawn my circle, and I only wish I knew at what point upon it the folk that we are in search of are to be found."

"I think I could lay my finger on it," said Holmes quietly.

"Really, now!" cried the inspector, "you have formed your opinion! Come, now, we shall see who agrees with you. I say it is south, for the country is more deserted there."

"And I say east," said my patient.

Ponderous - *Heavy, massive*
Overhauled – *Repaired*
Ordnance – *Weapons, Camon or Artillery*

"I am for west," remarked the plain-clothes man. "There are several quiet little villages up there." "And I am for north," said I, "because there are no hills there, and our friend says that he did not notice the carriage go up any."

"Come," cried the inspector, laughing; "it's a very pretty diversity of opinion. We have boxed the compass among us. Who do you give your casting vote to?"

"You are all wrong."

"But we can't all be."

"Oh, yes, you can. This is my point." He placed his finger in the centre of the circle. "This is where we shall find them."

"But the twelve-mile drive?" gasped Hatherley.

"Six out and six back. Nothing simpler. You say yourself that the horse was fresh and glossy when you got in. How could it be that if it had gone twelve miles over heavy roads?" "Indeed, it is a likely **ruse** enough," observed Bradstreet thoughtfully. "Of course, there can be no doubt as to the nature of this gang."

"None at all," said Holmes. "They are coiners on a large scale, and have used the machine to form the *amalgam* which has taken the place of silver."

"We have known for some time that a clever gang was at work," said the inspector. "They have been turning out half-crowns by the thousand. We even traced them as far as Reading, but could get no farther, for they had covered their traces in a way that showed that they were very old hands. But now, thanks to this lucky chance, I think that we have got them right enough."

But the inspector was mistaken, for those criminals were not destined to fall into the hands of justice. As we rolled into Eyford Station, we saw a gigantic column of smoke which streamed up from behind a small *clump* of trees in the neighbourhood and hung like an immense ostrich feather over the landscape.

"A house on fire?" asked Bradstreet as the train steamed off again on its way.

"Yes, sir!" said the station-master.

"When did it break out?"

"I hear that it was during the night, sir, but it has got worse, and the whole place is in a blaze."

"Whose house is it?"

"Dr. Becher's."

Inexorable –
Unavoidable
Ruse – *Trick*

Greatest   Adventure   Stories   of   Sherloc

"Tell me," broke in the engineer, "is Dr. Becher a German, very thin, with a long, sharp nose?" The station-master laughed heartily. "No, sir, Dr. Becher is an Englishman, and there isn't a man in the parish who has a better-lined waistcoat. But he has a gentleman staying with him, a patient, as I understand, who is a foreigner, and he looks as if a little good Berkshire beef would do him no harm."

The station-master had not finished his speech before we were all hastening in the direction of the fire. The road topped a low hill, and there was a great widespread whitewashed building in front of us, spouting fire at every *chink* and window, while in the garden in front, three fire-engines were vainly striving to keep the flames under.

"That's it!" cried Hatherley, in intense excitement. "There is the gravel-drive, and there are the rose-bushes where I lay. That second window is the one that I jumped from."

"Well, at least," said Holmes, "you have had your revenge upon them. There can be no question that it was your oil-lamp which, when it was crushed in the press, set fire to the wooden walls, though no doubt they were too excited in the chase after you to observe it at the time. Now keep your eyes open in this crowd for your friends of last night, though I very much fear that they are a good hundred miles off by now."

And Holmes's fears came to be realised, for from that day to this, no word has ever been heard either of the beautiful woman, the *sinister* German, or the morose Englishman. Early that morning, a peasant had met a cart containing several people and some very bulky boxes driving rapidly in the direction of Reading, but there all traces of the *fugitives* disappeared, and even Holmes's *ingenuity* failed ever to discover the least clue as to their whereabouts.

The firemen had been much **perturbed** at the strange arrangements which they had found within, and still more so by discovering a newly severed human thumb upon a window-sill of the second floor. About sunset, however, their efforts were at last successful, and they subdued the flames, but not before the roof had fallen in, and the whole place been reduced to such absolute ruin that, save some twisted cylinders and iron piping, not a trace remained of the machinery which had cost our unfortunate acquaintance so dearly. Large masses of nickel and of tin were discovered stored in an **out-house**, but no coins were

Chink - *A narrow opening*
Sinister - *Bad, evil, wicked*
Clump – *Bunch*

to be found, which may have explained the presence of those bulky boxes which have been already referred to.

How our hydraulic engineer had been conveyed from the garden to the spot, where he recovered his senses might have remained forever a mystery were it not for the soft mould, which told us a very plain tale. He had evidently been carried down by two persons, one of whom had remarkably small feet and the other unusually large ones. On the whole, it was most probable that the silent Englishman, being less bold or less murderous than his companion, had assisted the woman to bear the unconscious man out of the way of danger.

"Well," said our engineer *ruefully* as we took our seats to return once more to London, "it has been a pretty business for me! I have lost my thumb and I have lost a fifty-guinea fee, and what have I gained?"

"Experience," said Holmes, laughing. "Indirectly it may be of value, you know; you have only to put it into words to gain the reputation of being excellent company for the remainder of your existence."

Food For Thought

"Very well, said he, 'you shall know all about the machine'. Who said these words to whom, and what followed this event? Had the narrator not ultered the above words, what would have happened?

Bulky - *Very large size*
Perturbed - *Made uneasy or anxious*
Ruefully - *Feeling or expressing sorrow, or regret*
Fugitives – *Escapees*
Ingenuity – *Creativity*

An Understanding

Q. 1. What were the two cases that Watson brought to the notice of Sherlock Holmes?
Ans. _____
_____
_____
_____
_____

Q. 2. Why was Mr. Hatherley so keen or taking up the assignment of Colonel Lysander Stark?
Ans. _____
_____
_____
_____
_____

Q. 3. "How would fifty guineas for a night's work suit you?" Who said these words and to whom? Why were these words spoken?
Ans. _____
_____
_____
_____
_____

Q. 4. Why did Colonel Lysander Stark require a hydraulic engineer like Mr. Hatherley? What happened when Hatherley reached the destination as directed by the colonel?
Ans. _____
_____
_____
_____

The Adventure of the Empty House

~ Arthur Conan Doyle

IT was in the spring of the year, 1894 that all London was interested, and the fashionable world dismayed, by the murder of the Honourable Ronald Adair under most unusual and *inexplicable* circumstances. The public has already learnt those particulars of the crime which came out in the police investigation, but a good deal was suppressed upon that occasion, since the case for the prosecution was so overwhelmingly strong that it was not necessary to bring forward all the facts. Only now, at the end of nearly ten years, am I allowed to supply those missing links which make up the whole of that remarkable chain. The crime was of interest in itself, but that interest was as nothing to me compared to the inconceivable sequel, which afforded me the greatest shock and surprise of any event in my adventurous life. Even now, after this long interval, I find myself thrilling as I think of it, and feeling once more that sudden flood of joy, amazement, and *incredulity* which utterly submerged my mind. Let me say to that public, which has shown some interest in those glimpses which I have occasionally given them of the thoughts and actions of a very remarkable man, that they are not to blame me if I have not shared my knowledge with them, for I should have considered it my first duty to do so, had I not been barred by a positive prohibition from his own lips, which was only withdrawn upon the third of last month. It can be imagined that my close intimacy with Sherlock Holmes had interested me deeply in crime, and that after his disappearance, I never failed to read with care the various problems which came before the public. And I even attempted, more than once, for my own private satisfaction, to employ his methods in their solution, though with indifferent success. There was none, however, which appealed to me like this tragedy of Ronald Adair. As I read the evidence at the *inquest*, which led up to a verdict of wilful murder against some person or persons unknown, I realized more clearly than I had ever done the loss which the community had sustained by the death of Sherlock Holmes.

Inexplicable -
Unaccountable
Incredulity –
Disbelief
Inquest –
Investigation

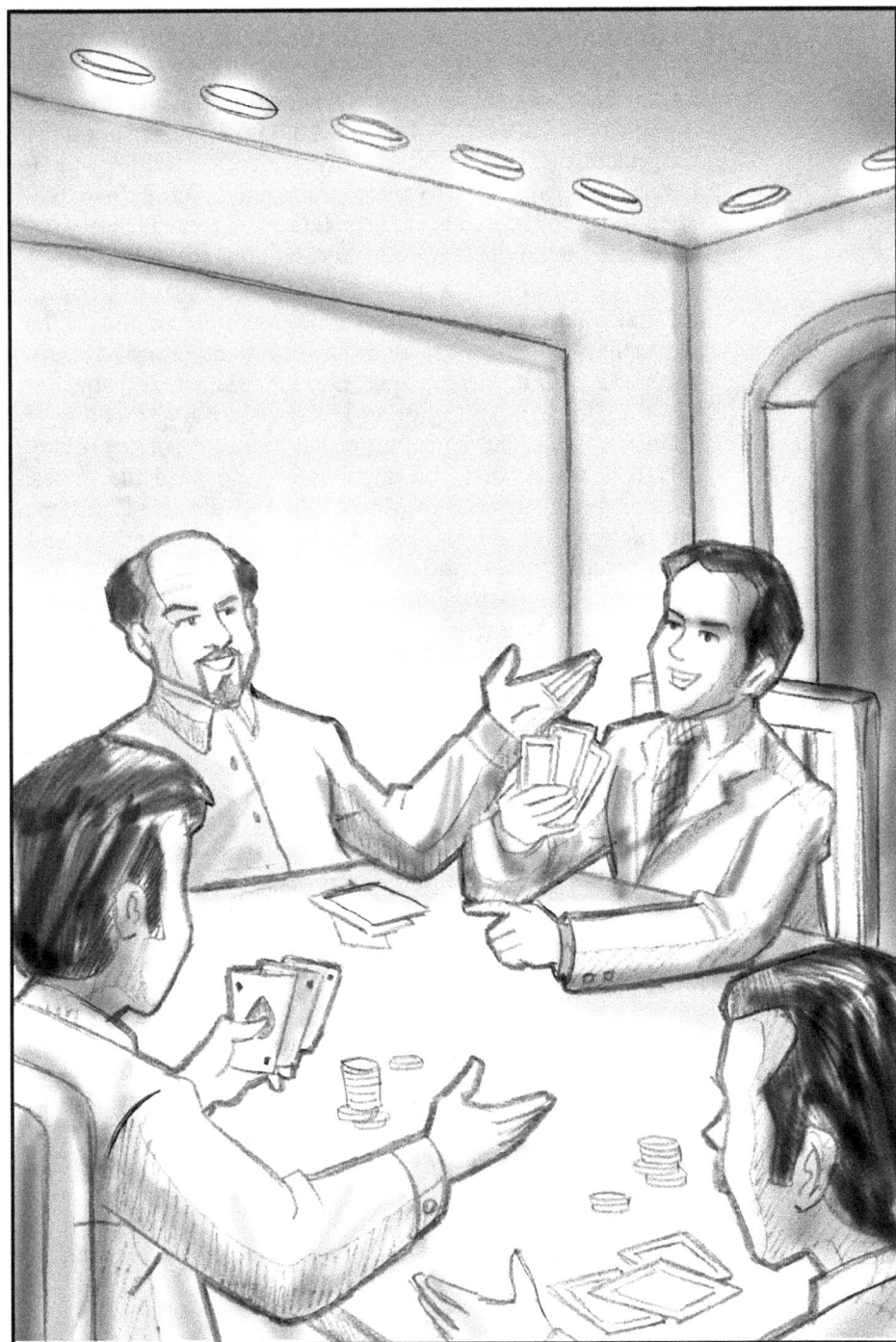

There were points about this strange business which would, I was sure, have specially appealed to him, and the efforts of the police would have been supplemented, or more probably, **anticipated**, by the trained observation and the alert mind of the first criminal agent in Europe. All day, as I drove upon my round, I turned over the case in my mind and found no explanation which appeared to me to be adequate. At the risk of telling a twice-told tale, I will **recapitulate** the facts as they were known to the public at the conclusion of the **inquest**.

The Honourable Ronald Adair was the second son of the Earl of Maynooth, at that time governor of one of the Australian colonies. Adair's mother had returned from Australia to undergo the operation for cataract, and she, her son Ronald, and her daughter Hilda were living together at 427 Park Lane. The youth moved in the best society – had, so far as was known, no enemies and no particular vices. He had been engaged to Miss Edith Woodley, of Carstairs, but the engagement had been broken off by mutual consent some months before, and there was no sign that it had left any very profound feeling behind it. For the rest {sic} the man's life moved in a narrow and conventional circle, for his habits were quiet and his nature unemotional. Yet it was upon this easy-going young aristocrat that death came, in most strange and unexpected form, between the hours of ten and eleven-twenty on the night of March 30, 1894.

Ronald Adair was fond of cards – playing continually, but never for such stakes as would hurt him. He was a member of the Baldwin, the Cavendish, and the Bagatelle card clubs. It was shown that, after dinner on the day of his death, he had played a rubber of **whist** at the latter club. He had also played there in the afternoon. The evidence of those who had played with him – Mr. Murray, Sir John Hardy, and Colonel Moran – showed that the game was whist, and that there was a fairly equal fall of the cards. Adair might have lost five pounds, but not more. His fortune was a considerable one, and such a loss could not in any way affect him. He had played nearly every day at one club or other, but he was a cautious player, and usually rose a winner. It came out in evidence that, in partnership with Colonel Moran, he had actually won as much as four hundred and twenty pounds in a sitting, some weeks before, from Godfrey Milner and Lord Balmoral. So much for his recent history as it came out at the inquest.

Recapitulate – *Sum up*
Anticipated - *Expected*
Inquest - *A legal or judicial inquiry*
Whist – *An English card game*

Greatest   Adventure   Stories   of   Sherloc

On the evening of the crime, he returned from the club exactly at ten. His mother and sister were out spending the evening with a relation. The servant *deposed* that she heard him enter the front room on the second floor, generally used as his sitting room. She had lit a fire there, and as it smoked, she had opened the window. No sound was heard from the room until eleven-twenty, the hour of the return of Lady Maynooth and her daughter. Desiring to say good-night, she attempted to enter her son's room. The door was locked on the inside, and no answer could be got to their cries and knocking. Help was obtained, and the door forced. The unfortunate young man was found lying near the table. His head had been horribly *mutilated* by an expanding revolver bullet, but no weapon of any sort was to be found in the room. On the table, lay two banknotes for ten pounds each and seventeen pounds, ten in silver and gold, the money arranged in little piles of varying amount. There were some figures also upon a sheet of paper, with the names of some club friends opposite to them, from which it was *conjectured* that before his death, he was endeavouring to make out his losses or winnings at cards.

A minute examination of the circumstances served only to make the case more complex. In the first place, no reason could be given why the young man should have fastened the door upon the inside. There was the possibility that the murderer had done this, and had afterwards escaped by the window. The drop was at least twenty feet, however, and a bed of *crocuses* in full bloom lay beneath. Neither the flowers nor the earth showed any sign of having been disturbed, nor were there any marks upon the narrow strip of grass which separated the house from the road. Apparently, therefore, it was the young man himself who had fastened the door. But how did he come by his death? No one could have climbed up to the window without leaving traces. Suppose a man had fired through the window, he would indeed be a remarkable shot who could with a revolver *inflict* so deadly a wound. Again, Park Lane is a frequented thoroughfare; there is a cab stand within a hundred yards of the house. No one had heard a shot. And yet there was the dead man and there the revolver bullet, which had mushroomed out, as soft-nosed bullets will, and so inflicted a wound which must have caused instantaneous death. Such were the circumstances of the Park Lane Mystery,

Conjectured - *Formation of an opinion*
Inflict - *To impose*
Mutilated - *To injure*
Deposed – *Removed*
Crocuses – *Types of bulb flower*

which were further complicated by entire absence of motive, since, as I have said, young Adair was not known to have any enemy, and no attempt had been made to remove the money or valuables in the room.

All day I turned these facts over in my mind, endeavouring to hit upon some theory which could reconcile them all, and to find that line of least resistance which my poor friend had declared to be the starting-point of every investigation. I confess that I made little progress. In the evening, I strolled across the Park, and found myself about six o'clock at the Oxford Street end of Park Lane. A group of *loafers* upon the pavements, all staring up at a particular window, directed me to the house which I had come to see. A tall, thin man with coloured glasses, whom I strongly suspected of being a plain-clothes detective, was pointing out some theory of his own, while the others crowded around to listen to what he said. I got as near him as I could, but his observations seemed to me to be absurd, so I withdrew again in some disgust. As I did so, I struck against an elderly, deformed man, who had been behind me, and I knocked down several books which he was carrying. I remember that as I picked them up, I observed the title of one of them, THE ORIGIN OF TREE WORSHIP, and it struck me that the fellow must be some poor *bibliophile*, who, either as a trade or as a hobby, was a collector of obscure volumes. I endeavoured to apologise for the accident, but it was evident that these books which I had so unfortunately maltreated were very precious objects in the eyes of their owner. With a snarl of contempt, he turned upon his heel, and I saw his curved back and white side-whiskers disappear among the *throng*.

My observations of No. 427 Park Lane did little to clear up the problem in which I was interested. The house was separated from the street by a low wall and railing, the whole not more than five feet high. It was perfectly easy, therefore, for anyone to get into the garden, but the window was entirely inaccessible, since there was no waterpipe or anything which could help the most active man to climb it. More puzzled than ever, I retraced my steps to Kensington. I had not been in my study five minutes when the maid entered to say that a person desired to see me. To my astonishment, it was none other than my strange old book collector, his sharp, **wizened** face peering out from a frame of

Bibliophile – *One who loves to read and collect books*
Throng - *Assembled together*
Loafers - *Idlers*
Wizened – *Aged*

white hair, and his precious volumes, a dozen of them at least, *wedged* under his right arm.

"You're surprised to see me, sir," said he, in a strange, croaking voice.

I acknowledged that I was.

"Well, I've a conscience, sir, and when I chanced to see you go into this house, as I came *hobbling* after you, I thought to myself, I'll just step in and see that kind gentleman, and tell him that if I was a bit *gruff* in my manner, but there was not any harm meant, and that I am much obliged to him for picking up my books."

"You make too much of a trifle," said I. "May I ask how you knew who I was?"

"Well, sir, if it isn't too great a liberty, I am a neighbour of yours, for you'll find my little bookshop at the corner of Church Street, and very happy to see you, I am sure. Maybe you collect yourself, sir. Here's BRITISH BIRDS, and CATULLUS, and THE HOLY WAR – a bargain, every one of them. With five volumes, you could just fill that gap on that second shelf. It looks untidy, does it not, sir?"

I moved my head to look at the cabinet behind me. When I turned again, Sherlock Holmes was standing smiling at me across my study table. I rose to my feet, stared at him for some seconds in utter amazement, and then it appeared that I must have fainted for the first and the last time in my life. Certainly a grey mist swirled before my eyes, and when it cleared, I found my collar-ends undone and the tingling after-taste of brandy upon my lips. Holmes was bending over my chair, his flask in his hand.

"My dear Watson," said the well-remembered voice, "I owe you a thousand apologies. I had no idea that you would be so affected."

I gripped him by the arms.

"Holmes!" I cried. "Is it really you? Can it indeed be that you are alive? Is it possible that you succeeded in climbing out of that awful *abyss*?"

"Wait a moment," said he. "Are you sure that you are really fit to discuss things? I have given you a serious shock by my unnecessarily dramatic reappearance."

"I am all right, but indeed, Holmes, I can hardly believe my eyes. Good heavens! to think that you – you of all men

Wedged – *Stuck*
Abyss - *A deep space gulf or cavity*
Gruff - *Hoarse*
Hobbling – *Limping*

– should be standing in my study." Again I gripped him by the sleeve, and felt the thin, *sinewy* arm beneath it. "Well, you're not a spirit anyhow," said I. "My dear chap, I'm overjoyed to see you. Sit down, and tell me how you came alive out of that dreadful *chasm*."

He sat opposite to me, and lit a cigarette in his old, *non-chalant* manner. He was dressed in the *seedy* frockcoat of the book merchant, but the rest of that individual lay in a pile of white hair and old books upon the table. Holmes looked even thinner and keener than of old, but there was a dead-white tinge in his *aquiline* face which told me that his life recently had not been a healthy one.

"I am glad to stretch myself, Watson," said he. "It is no joke when a tall man has to take a foot off his stature for several hours on end. Now, my dear fellow, in the matter of these explanations, we have, if I may ask for your cooperation, a hard and dangerous night's work in front of us. Perhaps, it would be better if I gave you an account of the whole situation when that work is finished."

"I am full of curiosity. I should much prefer to hear now."

"You'll come with me tonight?"

"When you like and where you like."

"This is, indeed, like the old days. We shall have time for a mouthful of dinner before we need go. Well, then, about that chasm. I had no serious difficulty in getting out of it, for the very simple reason that I never was in it."

"You never were in it?"

"No, Watson, I never was in it. My note to you was absolutely genuine. I had little doubt that I had come to the end of my career when I perceived the somewhat *sinister* figure of the late Professor Moriarty standing upon the narrow pathway which led to safety. I read an *inexorable* purpose in his grey eyes. I exchanged some remarks with him, therefore, and obtained his courteous permission to write the short note which you afterwards received. I left it with my cigarette-box and my stick, and I walked along the pathway, Moriarty still at my heels. When I reached the end, I stood at bay. He drew no weapon, but he rushed at me and threw his long arms around me. He knew that his own game was up, and was only anxious to revenge himself upon me. We tottered together upon

Chasm - *A gorge*
Aquiline - *Hooked*
Non-chalant - *Unconcerned*
Sinister - *Bad, evil*
Inexorable - *Unyielding*
Sinewy – *Lean and strong*
Seedy – *Sordid*

Greatest   Adventure   Stories   of   Sherloc

the brink of the fall. I have some knowledge, however, of *baritsu*, or the Japanese system of wrestling, which has more than once been very useful to me. I slipped through his grip, and he with a horrible scream kicked madly for a few seconds, and clawed the air with both his hands. But for all his efforts, he could not get his balance, and over he went. With my face over the **brink**, I saw him fall for a long way. Then he struck a rock, bounded off, and splashed into the water."

I listened with amazement to this explanation, which Holmes delivered between the puffs of his cigarette.

"But the tracks!" I cried. "I saw, with my own eyes, that the two went down the path and none returned."

"It came about in this way. The instant that the Professor had disappeared, it struck me what a really extraordinarily lucky chance Fate had placed in my way. I knew that Moriarty was not the only man who had sworn my death. There were at least three others whose desire for vengeance upon me would only be increased by the death of their leader. They were all most dangerous men. One or other would certainly get me. On the other hand, if all the world was convinced that I was dead, they would take liberties, these men, they would soon lay themselves open, and sooner or later, I could destroy them. Then it would be time for me to announce that I was still in the land of the living. So rapidly does the brain act that I believe I had thought this all out before Professor Moriarty had reached the bottom of the Reichenbach Fall.

"I stood up and examined the rocky wall behind me. In your picturesque account of the matter, which I read with great interest some months later, you assert that the wall was sheer. That was not literally true. A few small footholds presented themselves, and there was some indication of a **ledge**. The cliff is so high that to climb it all was an obvious impossibility, and it was equally impossible to make my way along the wet path without leaving some tracks. I might, it is true, have reversed my boots, as I have done on similar occasions, but the sight of three sets of tracks in one direction would certainly have suggested a **deception**. On the whole, then, it was best that I should risk the climb. It was not a pleasant business, Watson. The fall roared beneath me. I am not a fanciful person, but I give you my word that I seemed to hear Moriarty's voice screaming at me out of the abyss. A mistake would have been fatal. More than once, as **tufts** of grass came out in my hand or

Deception - *Fraudulence*

Brink - *An extreme edge, Verge*

Ledge – *Shelf*

Tufts – *Bunches*

my foot slipped in the wet notches of the rock, I thought that I was gone. But I struggled upward, and at last I reached a ledge several feet deep and covered with soft green moss, where I could lie unseen, in the most perfect comfort. There I was stretched, when you, my dear Watson, and all your following were investigating in the most sympathetic and inefficient manner the circumstances of my death.

"At last, when you had all formed your inevitable and totally *erroneous* conclusions, you departed for the hotel, and I was left alone. I had imagined that I had reached the end of my adventures, but a very unexpected occurrence showed me that there were surprises still in store for me. A huge rock, falling from above, boomed past me, struck the path, and bounded over into the chasm. For an instant, I thought that it was an accident, but a moment later, looking up, I saw a man's head against the darkening sky, and another stone struck the very ledge upon which I was stretched, within a foot of my head. Of course, the meaning of this was obvious. Moriarty had not been alone. A *confederate* – and even that one glance had told me how dangerous a man that confederate was – had kept guard while the Professor had attacked me. From a distance, unseen by me, he had been a witness of his friend's death and of my escape. He had waited, and then making his way around to the top of the cliff, he had endeavoured to succeed where his comrade had failed.

"I did not take long to think about it, Watson. Again I saw that grim face look over the cliff, and I knew that it was the *precursor* of another stone. I scrambled down on to the path. I don't think I could have done it in cold blood. It was a hundred times more difficult than getting up. But I had no time to think of the danger, for another stone sang past me as I hung by my hands from the edge of the ledge. Halfway down I slipped, but, by the blessing of God, I landed, torn and bleeding, upon the path. I took to my heels, did ten miles over the mountains in the darkness, and a week later, I found myself in Florence, with the certainty that no one in the world knew what had become of me.

"I had only one *confidant* – my brother Mycroft. I owe you many apologies, my dear Watson, but it was all-important that it should be thought I was dead, and it is quite certain that you would not have written so convincing an account of my unhappy end had you not yourself thought that it was

Confederate -
Alliance
Erroneous –
Mistaken
Confidant – *One to whom secrets are disclosed*
Precursor - *A person or thing that precedes*

Greatest   Adventure   Stories   of   Sherloc

true. Several times during the last three years I have taken up my pen to write to you, but always I feared lest your affectionate regard for me should tempt you to some *indiscretion* which would betray my secret. For that reason, I turned away from you this evening, when you upset my books, for I was in danger at the time, and any show of surprise and emotion upon your part might have drawn attention to my identity and led to the most *deplorable* and irreparable results. As to Mycroft, I had to confide in him in order to obtain the money which I needed. The course of events in London did not run so well as I had hoped, for the trial of the Moriarty gang left two of its most dangerous members, my own most *vindictive* enemies, at liberty. I travelled for two years in Tibet, therefore, and amused myself by visiting Lhassa, and spending some days with the head lama. You may have read of the remarkable explorations of a Norwegian named Sigerson, but I am sure that it never occurred to you that you were receiving news of your friend. I then passed through Persia, looked in at Mecca, and paid a short but interesting visit to the Khalifa at Khartoum, the results of which I have communicated to the Foreign Office. Returning to France, I spent some months in a research into the coal-tar derivatives, which I conducted in a laboratory at Montpellier, in the south of France. Having concluded this to my satisfaction and learning that only one of my enemies was now left in London, I was about to return when my movements were hastened by the news of this very remarkable Park Lane Mystery, which not only appealed to me by its own merits, but which seemed to offer some most peculiar personal opportunities. I came over at once to London, called in my own person at Baker Street, threw Mrs. Hudson into violent hysterics, and found that Mycroft had preserved my rooms and my papers exactly as they had always been. So it was, my dear Watson, that at two o'clock today, I found myself in my old armchair in my own old room, and only wishing that I could have seen my old friend Watson in the other chair which he has so often adorned."

Such was the remarkable narrative to which I listened on that April evening – a narrative which would have been utterly incredible to me had it not been confirmed by the actual sight of the tall, spare figure and the keen, eager face, which I had never thought to see again. In some manner, he had learned of my own sad *bereavement*, and his sympathy was shown in his

Indiscretion - *Imprudence*
Deplorable - *Lamentable*
Vindictive – *Spiteful*
Bereavement – *Grief*

manner rather than in his words. "Work is the best *antidote* to sorrow, my dear Watson," said he; "and I have a piece of work for us both tonight which, if we can bring it to a successful conclusion, will in itself justify a man's life on this planet." In vain, I begged him to tell me more. "You will hear and see enough before morning," he answered. "We have three years of the past to discuss. Let that suffice until half-past nine, when we start upon the notable adventure of the empty house."

It was indeed like old times when, at that hour, I found myself seated beside him in a hansom, my revolver in my pocket, and the thrill of adventure in my heart. Holmes was cold and stern and silent. As the gleam of the street-lamps flashed upon his *austere* features, I saw that his brows were drawn down in thought and his thin lips compressed. I knew not what wild beast we were about to hunt down in the dark jungle of criminal London, but I was well assured, from the bearing of this master huntsman, that the adventure was a most grave one – while the *sardonic* smile which occasionally broke through his ascetic gloom boded little good for the object of our quest.

I had imagined that we were bound for Baker Street, but Holmes stopped the cab at the corner of Cavendish Square. I observed that as he stepped out he gave a most searching glance to right and left, and at every subsequent street corner, he took the utmost pains to assure that he was not followed. Our route was certainly a singular one. Holmes's knowledge of the byways of London was extraordinary, and on this occasion, he passed rapidly and with an assured step through a network of *mews* and stables, the very existence of which I had never known. We emerged at last into a small road, lined with old, gloomy houses, which led us into Manchester Street, and so to Blandford Street. Here he turned swiftly down a narrow passage, passed through a wooden gate into a deserted yard, and then opened with a key the back door of a house. We entered together, and he closed it behind us.

The place was pitch dark, but it was evident to me that it was an empty house. Our feet creaked and crackled over the bare planking, and my outstretched hand touched a wall from which the paper was hanging in ribbons. Holmes's cold, thin fingers closed around my wrist and led me forward down a long hall, until I dimly saw the *murky* fanlight over the door. Here Holmes turned suddenly to the right and we found

Murky - *Dark, Gloomy*
Mews - *A row of stables*
Boded - *To be an omen of*
Antidote - *A medicine or remedy*
Austere – *Severe*
Sardonic – *Sarcastic*

ourselves in a large, square, empty room, heavily shadowed in the corners, but faintly lit in the centre from the lights of the street beyond. There was no lamp near, and the window was thick with dust, so that we could only just *discern* each other's figures within. My companion put his hand upon my shoulder and his lips close to my ear.

"Do you know where we are?" he whispered.

"Surely that is Baker Street" I answered, staring through the dim window.

"Exactly. We are in Camden House, which stands opposite to our own old quarters."

"But why are we here?"

"Because it commands so excellent a view of that *picturesque* pile. Might I trouble you, my dear Watson, to draw a little nearer to the window, taking every precaution not to show yourself, and then to look up at our old rooms – the starting point of so many of your little fairy tales? We will see if my three years of absence have entirely taken away my power to surprise you."

I crept forward and looked across at the familiar window. As my eyes fell upon it, I gave a gasp and a cry of amazement. The blind was down, and a strong light was burning in the room. The shadow of a man who was seated in a chair within was thrown in hard, black outline upon the luminous screen of the window. There was no mistaking the *poise* of the head, the squareness of the shoulders, the sharpness of the features. The face was turned half-round, and the effect was that of one of those black silhouettes which our grandparents loved to frame. It was a perfect reproduction of Holmes. So amazed was I that I threw out my hand to make sure that the man himself was standing beside me. He was quivering with silent laughter.

"Well?" said he.

"Good heavens!" I cried. "It is marvellous."

"I trust that age doth not wither nor custom stale my infinite variety," said he, and I recognised in his voice the joy and pride which the artist takes in his own creation. "It really is rather like me, is it not?"

"I should be prepared to swear that it was you."

"The credit of the execution is due to Monsieur Oscar Meunier, of Grenoble, who spent some days in doing the

Discern - *Apprehend*
Picturesque – *Scenic*
Poise – *Composure*

moulding. It is a bust in wax. The rest I arranged myself during my visit to Baker Street this afternoon."

"But why?"

"Because, my dear Watson, I had the strongest possible reason for wishing certain people to think that I was there when I was really elsewhere."

"And you thought the rooms were watched?"

"I KNEW that they were watched."

"By whom?"

"By my old enemies, Watson. By the charming society whose leader lies in the Reichenbach Fall. You must remember that they knew, and only they knew, that I was still alive. Sooner or later, they believed that I should come back to my rooms. They watched them continuously, and this morning they saw me arrive."

"How do you know?"

"Because I recognised their *sentinel* when I glanced out of my window. He is a harmless enough fellow, Parker by name, a *garroter* by trade, and a remarkable performer upon the jew's-harp. I cared nothing for him. But I cared a great deal for the much more formidable person who was behind him, the bosom friend of Moriarty, the man who dropped the rocks over the cliff, the most cunning and dangerous criminal in London. That is the man who is after me tonight Watson, and that is the man who is quite unaware that we are after him."

My friend's plans were gradually revealing themselves. From this convenient retreat, the watchers were being watched and the trackers tracked. That angular shadow up yonder was the bait, and we were the hunters. In silence, we stood together in the darkness and watched the hurrying figures who passed and repassed in front of us. Holmes was silent and motionless; but I could tell that he was keenly alert, and that his eyes were fixed intently upon the stream of passers-by. It was a bleak and *boisterous* night and the wind whistled shrilly down the long street. Many people were moving to and fro, most of them muffled in their coats and *cravats*. Once or twice, it seemed to me that I had seen the same figure before, and I especially noticed two men who appeared to be sheltering themselves from the wind in the doorway of a house some distance up the street. I tried to draw my companion's attention to them; but he gave a little ejaculation of impatience, and continued

Cravats - *Neckties*
Boisterous - *Rough ad noisy*
Sentinel – *Guard*
Garroter – *Executer*

Greatest   Adventure   Stories   of   Sherloc

to stare into the street. More than once, he *fidgeted* with his feet and tapped rapidly with his fingers upon the wall. It was evident to me that he was becoming uneasy, and that his plans were not working out altogether as he had hoped. At last, as midnight approached and the street gradually cleared, he paced up and down the room in uncontrollable agitation. I was about to make some remark to him, when I raised my eyes to the lighted window, and again experienced almost as great a surprise as before. I clutched Holmes's arm, and pointed upward.

"The shadow has moved!" I cried.

It was indeed no longer the profile, but the back, which was turned towards us.

Three years had certainly not smoothed the *asperities* of his temper or his impatience with a less active intelligence than his own.

"Of course it has moved," said he. "Am I such a *farcical* bungler, Watson, that I should erect an obvious dummy, and expect that some of the sharpest men in Europe would be deceived by it? We have been in this room two hours, and Mrs. Hudson has made some change in that figure eight times, or once in every quarter of an hour. She works it from the front, so that her shadow may never be seen. Ah!" He drew in his breath with a shrill, excited intake. In the dim light, I saw his head thrown forward, his whole attitude rigid with attention. Outside the street was absolutely deserted. Those two men might still be crouching in the doorway, but I could no longer see them. All was still and dark, save only that brilliant yellow screen in front of us with the black figure outlined upon its centre. Again in the utter silence, I heard that thin, *sibilant* note which spoke of intense suppressed excitement. An instant later, he pulled me back into the blackest corner of the room, and I felt his warning hand upon my lips. The fingers which clutched me were quivering. Never had I known my friend more moved, and yet the dark street still stretched lonely and motionless before us.

But suddenly I was aware of that which his keener senses had already distinguished. A low, *stealthy* sound came to my ears, not from the direction of Baker Street, but from the back of the very house in which we lay concealed. A door opened and shut. An instant later, steps crept down the passage – steps which were meant to be silent, but which *reverberated* harshly

Stealthy - *Furtive*
Sibilant - *Hissing sound*
Fidgeted - *Made uneasy*
Reverberated - *Recoiled, Rebounded*
Asperities – *Hardships*
Farcical – *Absurd*

through the empty house. Holmes crouched back against the wall, and I did the same, my hand closing upon the handle of my revolver. Peering through the gloom, I saw the vague outline of a man, a shade blacker than the blackness of the open door. He stood for an instant, and then he crept forward, crouching, *menacing*, into the room. He was within three yards of us, this sinister figure, and I had braced myself to meet his spring, before I realised that he had no idea of our presence. He passed close beside us, stole over to the window, and very softly and noiselessly raised it for half a foot. As he sank to the level of this opening, the light of the street, no longer dimmed by the dusty glass, fell full upon his face. The man seemed to be beside himself with excitement. His two eyes shone like stars, and his features were working *convulsively*. He was an elderly man, with a thin, projecting nose, a high, bald forehead, and a huge grizzled moustache. An opera hat was pushed to the back of his head, and an evening dress shirt-front gleamed out through his open overcoat. His face was *gaunt* and *swarthy*, scored with deep, savage lines. In his hand, he carried what appeared to be a stick, but as he laid it down upon the floor it gave a metallic clang. Then from the pocket of his overcoat, he drew a bulky object, and he busied himself in some task which ended with a loud, sharp click, as if a spring or bolt had fallen into its place. Still kneeling upon the floor, he bent forward and threw all his weight and strength upon some lever, with the result that there came a long, whirling, grinding noise, ending once more in a powerful click. He straightened himself then, and I saw that what he held in his hand was a sort of gun, with a curiously misshapen butt. He opened it at the breech, put something in, and snapped the breech-lock. Then, crouching down, he rested the end of the barrel upon the ledge of the open window, and I saw his long moustache droop over the stock and his eye gleam as it peered along the sights. I heard a little sigh of satisfaction as he cuddled the butt into his shoulder; and saw that amazing target, the black man on the yellow ground, standing clear at the end of his foresight. For an instant, he was rigid and motionless. Then his finger tightened on the trigger. There was a strange, loud whiz and a long, silvery tinkle of broken glass. At that instant, Holmes sprang like a tiger on to the marksman's back, and hurled him flat upon his face. He was up again in a moment, and with convulsive strength, he seized Holmes by the throat, but I struck him on the head with the butt of my revolver,

Gaunt - *Extremely thin and bony*
Menacing - *Annoying*
Convulsively – *With spasms*
Swarthy – *Dark*

Greatest   Adventure   Stories   of   Sherloc

and he dropped again upon the floor. I fell upon him, and as I held him, my comrade blew a shrill call upon a whistle. There was the clatter of running feet upon the pavement, and two policemen in uniform, with one plain-clothes detective, rushed through the front entrance and into the room.

"That you, Lestrade?" said Holmes.

"Yes, Mr. Holmes. I took the job myself. It's good to see you back in London, sir."

"I think you want a little unofficial help. Three undetected murders in one year won't do, Lestrade. But you handled the Molesey Mystery with less than your usual – that's to say, you handled it fairly well."

We had all risen to our feet, our prisoner breathing hard, with a stalwart constable on each side of him. Already a few *loiterers* had begun to collect in the street. Holmes stepped up to the window, closed it, and dropped the blinds. Lestrade had produced two candles, and the policemen had uncovered their lanterns. I was able at last to have a good look at our prisoner.

It was a tremendously *virile* and yet sinister face which was turned towards us. With the brow of a philosopher above and the jaw of a sensualist below, the man must have started with great capacities for good or for evil. But one could not look upon his cruel blue eyes, with their drooping, cynical lids, or upon the fierce, aggressive nose and the threatening, deep-lined brow, without reading Nature's plainest danger-signals. He took no heed of any of us, but his eyes were fixed upon Holmes's face with an expression in which hatred and amazement were equally blended. "You *fiend*!" he kept on muttering. "You clever, clever fiend!"

"Ah, Colonel!" said Holmes, arranging his rumpled collar. "'Journeys end in lovers' meetings,' as the old play says. I don't think I have had the pleasure of seeing you since you favoured me with those attentions as I lay on the ledge above the Reichenbach Fall."

The colonel still stared at my friend like a man in a trance. "You cunning, cunning fiend!" was all that he could say.

"I have not introduced you yet," said Holmes. "This, gentlemen, is Colonel Sebastian Moran, once of Her Majesty's Indian Army, and the best heavy-game shot that our Eastern Empire has ever produced. I believe I am correct Colonel, in saying that your bag of tigers still remains unrivalled?"

Loiterers - *Idlers*
Virile – *Having strength and energy*
Fiend – *Evil person*

The fierce old man said nothing, but still glared at my companion. With his savage eyes and bristling moustache he was wonderfully like a tiger himself.

"I wonder that my very simple *stratagem* could deceive so old a *shikari*," said Holmes. "It must be very familiar to you. Have you not *tethered* a young kid under a tree, lain above it with your rifle, and waited for the bait to bring up your tiger? This empty house is my tree, and you are my tiger. You have possibly had other guns in reserve in case there should be several tigers, or in the unlikely supposition of your own aim failing you. These," he pointed around, "are my other guns. The parallel is exact."

Colonel Moran sprang forward with a snarl of rage, but the constables dragged him back. The fury upon his face was terrible to look at.

"I confess that you had one small surprise for me," said Holmes. "I did not anticipate that you would yourself make use of this empty house and this convenient front window. I had imagined you as operating from the street, where my friend, Lestrade and his merry men were awaiting you. With that exception, all has gone as I expected."

Colonel Moran turned to the official detective.

"You may or may not have just cause for arresting me," said he, "but at least there can be no reason why I should submit to the *gibes* of this person. If I am in the hands of the law, let things be done in a legal way."

"Well, that's reasonable enough," said Lestrade. "Nothing further you have to say, Mr. Holmes, before we go?"

Holmes had picked up the powerful air-gun from the floor, and was examining its mechanism. "An admirable and unique weapon," said he, "noiseless and of tremendous power: I knew Von Herder, the blind German mechanic, who constructed it to the order of the late Professor Moriarty. For years, I have been aware of its existance though I have never before had the opportunity of handling it. I commend it very specially to your attention, Lestrade and also the bullets which fit it."

Gibes - *Mocking or scoffing words, jeer*
Stratagem – *Trick*
Tethered – *Tied to a place with a rope*

"You can trust us to look after that, Mr. Holmes," said Lestrade, as the whole party moved towards the door. "Anything further to say?"

"Only to ask what charge you intend to prefer?"

"What charge, sir? Why, of course, the attempted murder of Mr. Sherlock Holmes."

"Not so, Lestrade. I do not propose to appear in the matter at all. To you, and to you only, belongs the credit of the remarkable arrest which you have effected. Yes, Lestrade, I congratulate you! With your usual happy mixture of cunning and audacity, you have got him." "Got him! Got whom, Mr. Holmes?"

"The man that the whole force has been seeking in vain – Colonel Sebastian Moran, who shot the Honourable Ronald Adair with an expanding bullet from an air-gun through the open window of the second-floor front of No. 427 Park Lane, upon the thirtieth of last month. That's the charge, Lestrade. And now, Watson, if you can endure the draught from a broken window, I think that half an hour in my study over a cigar may afford you some profitable amusement."

Our old chambers had been left unchanged through the supervision of Mycroft Holmes and the immediate care of Mrs. Hudson. As I entered I saw, it is true, an *unwonted* tidiness, but the old landmarks were all in their place. There were the chemical corner and the acid-stained, deal-topped table. There upon a shelf was the row of formidable scrapbooks and books of reference which many of our fellow-citizens would have been so glad to burn. The diagrams, the violin-case, and the pipe-rack – even the Persian slipper which contained the tobacco – all met my eyes as I glanced around me. There were two occupants of the room – one, Mrs. Hudson, who beamed upon us both as we entered – the other, the strange dummy which had played so important a part in the evening's adventures. It was a wax-coloured model of my friend, so admirably done that it was a perfect *facsimile*. It stood on a small pedestal table with an old dressing-gown of Holmes's so draped around it that the illusion from the street was absolutely perfect.

"I hope you observed all precautions, Mrs. Hudson?" said Holmes.

"I went to it on my knees, sir, just as you told me."

"Excellent. You carried the thing out very well. Did you observe where the bullet went?"

"Yes, sir. I'm afraid it has spoilt your beautiful bust, for it passed right through the head and flattened itself on the wall. I picked it up from the carpet. Here it is!"

Unwonted – *Unusual*
Facsimile – *Exact copy*

Holmes held it out to me. "A soft revolver bullet, as you perceive, Watson. There's genius in that, for who would expect to find such a thing fired from an airgun? All right, Mrs. Hudson. I am much obliged for your assistance. And now, Watson, let me see you in your old seat once more, for there are several points which I should like to discuss with you."

He had thrown off the seedy frockcoat, and now he was the Holmes of old in the mouse-coloured dressing-gown which he took from his *effigy*.

"The old *shikari's* nerves have not lost their steadiness, nor his eyes their *keenness*," said he, with a laugh, as he inspected the shattered forehead of his bust.

"Plumb in the middle of the back of the head and smack through the brain. He was the best shot in India, and I expect that there are few better in London. Have you heard the name?"

"No, I have not."

"Well, well, such is fame! But, then, if I remember right, you had not heard the name of Professor James Moriarty, who had one of the great brains of the century. Just give me down my index of biographies from the shelf."

He turned over the pages lazily, leaning back in his chair and blowing great clouds from his cigar.

"My collection of M's is a fine one," said he. "Moriarty himself is enough to make any letter illustrious, and here is Morgan the poisoner, and Merridew of *abominable* memory, and Mathews, who knocked out my left canine in the waiting-room at Charing Cross, and, finally, here is our friend of to-night."

He handed over the book, and I read:

MORAN, SEBASTIAN, COLONEL. Unemployed. Formerly 1st Bangalore Pioneers. Born London, 1840. Son of Sir Augustus Moran, C. B., once British Minister to Persia. Educated Eton and Oxford. Served in Jowaki Campaign, Afghan Campaign, Charasiab (despatches), Sherpur, and Cabul. Author of HEAVY GAME OF THE WESTERN HIMALAYAS (1881); THREE MONTHS IN THE JUNGLE (1884). Address: Conduit Street. Clubs: The Anglo-Indian, the Tankerville, the Bagatelle Card Club.

On the margin was written, in Holmes's precise hand:

Abominable -
Detestable, Loathsome
Effigy – *Dummy or statue*
Keenness –
Eagerness

The second most dangerous man in London.

"This is astonishing," said I, as I handed back the volume. "The man's career is that of an honourable soldier."

"It is true," Holmes answered. "Up to a certain point, he did well. He was always a man of iron nerve, and the story is still told in India how he crawled down a drain after a wounded man-eating tiger. There are some trees, Watson, which grow to a certain height, and then suddenly develop some unsightly eccentricity. You will see it often in humans. I have a theory that the individual represents in his development the whole procession of his ancestors, and that such a sudden turn to good or evil stands for some strong influence which came into the line of his *pedigree*. The person becomes, as it were, the *epitome* of the history of his own family."

"It is surely rather fanciful."

"Well, I don't insist upon it. Whatever the cause, Colonel Moran began hot to hold him. He retired, came to London, and again acquired an evil name. It was at this time that he was sought out by Professor Moriarty, to whom for a time he was chief of the staff. Moriarty supplied him liberally with the money, and used him only in one or two very high-class jobs, which no ordinary criminal could have undertaken. You may have some recollection of the death of Mrs. Stewart, of Lauder, in 1887. Not? Well, I am sure Moran was at the bottom of it, but nothing could be proved. So cleverly was the colonel concealed that, even when the Moriarty gang was broken up, we could not *incriminate* him. You remember at that date, when I called upon you in your rooms, how I put up the shutters for fear of air-guns? No doubt you thought me fanciful. I knew exactly what I was doing, for I knew of the existence of this remarkable gun, and I knew also that one of the best shots in the world would be behind it. When we were in Switzerland he followed us with Moriarty, and it was undoubtedly he who gave me that evil five minutes on the Reichenbach ledge.

"You may think that I read the papers with some attention during my *sojourn* in France, on the look-out for any chance of laying him by the heels. So long as he was free in London, my life would really not have been worth living. Night and day, the shadow would have been over me, and sooner or later his chance must have come. What could I do? I could not shoot him at sight, or I should myself be in the dock. There was no use appealing to a magistrate. They cannot interfere on the

Incriminate - *To accuse of on present proof of a crime*
Pedigree - *Anestry*
Epitome – *Essence*
Sojourn – *Stopover*

strength of what would appear to them to be a wild suspicion. So I could do nothing. But I watched the criminal news, knowing that sooner or later, I should get him. Then came the death of this Ronald Adair. My chance had come at last. Knowing what I did, was it not certain that Colonel Moran had done it? He had played cards with the lad, he had followed him home from the club, he had shot him through the open window. There was not a doubt of it. The bullets alone are enough to put his head in a noose. I came over at once. I was seen by the *sentinel*, who would, I knew, direct the colonel's attention to my presence. He could not fail to connect my sudden return with his crime, and to be terribly alarmed. I was sure that he would make an attempt to get me out of the way AT once, and would bring, round his murderous weapon for that purpose. I left him an excellent mark in the window, and, having warned the police that they might be needed – by the way, Watson, you spotted their presence in that doorway with *unerring* accuracy – I took up what seemed to me to be a judicious post for observation, never dreaming that he would choose the same spot for his attack. Now, my dear Watson, does anything remain for me to explain?"

"Yes," said I. "You have not made it clear what was Colonel Moran's motive in murdering the Honourable Ronald Adair?"

"Ah! my dear Watson, there we come into those realms of *conjecture*, where the most logical mind may be at fault. Each may form his own hypothesis upon the present evidence, and yours is as likely to be correct as mine."

"You have formed one, then?"

"I think that it is not difficult to explain the facts. It came out in evidence that Colonel Moran and young Adair had, between them, won a considerable amount of money. Now, undoubtedly played foul – of that I have long been aware. I believe that on the day of the murder, Adair had discovered that Moran was cheating. Very likely he had spoken to him privately, and had threatened to expose him unless he voluntarily resigned his membership of the club, and promised not to play cards again. It is unlikely that a youngster like Adair would at once make a hideous scandal by exposing a well known man so much older than himself. Probably he acted as I suggest. The exclusion from his clubs would mean ruin to Moran, who lived by his ill-gotten card-gains. He therefore murdered Adair, who at the time was endeavouring to

Sentinel - *A soldier tationed as a guard*
Unerring - *Undeviatingly accurate*
Conjecture - *Guess, speculation*

work out how much money he should himself return, since he could not profit by his partner's foul play. He locked the door lest the ladies should surprise him and insist upon knowing what he was doing with these names and coins. Will it pass?"

"I have no doubt that you have hit upon the truth."

"It will be *verified* or disproved at the trial. Meanwhile, come what may, Colonel Moran will trouble us no more. The famous air-gun of Von Herder will *embellish* the Scotland Yard Museum, and once again Mr. Sherlock Holmes is free to devote his life to examining those interesting little problems which the complex life of London so plentifully presents."

Food For Thought

The circumstances of the 'Park Lane Mystery' were very complicated because of the absence of motive, since Ronald Adair neither had enemies, nor any money or valuables were lost from his room, where he lay dead. Why do you think was it so? What would have happened if Holmes wouldnot have taken up this case?

Verified – *Established*
Embellish – *Decorate*

An Understanding

Q. 1. Who was Ronald Adair? What was he fond of?
Ans. _____
_____
_____
_____
_____

Q. 2. What were the strange circumstances under which Ronald Adair was found dead in his room?
Ans. _____
_____
_____
_____
_____

Q. 3. How did Sherlock Holmes hide himself for three years and how did he reveal his identity before Dr. Watson?
Ans. _____
_____
_____
_____
_____

Q. 4. Colonel Moran ad Professor Moriarty were one and the same person. Prove the above statement by giving instances from the story.
Ans. _____
_____
_____
_____
_____

The Adventure of the Copper Beeches

– Arthur Conan Doyle

"To the man who loves art for its own sake," remarked Sherlock Holmes, tossing aside the advertisement sheet of the Daily *Telegraph*, "it is frequently in its least important and lowliest manifestations that the keenest pleasure is to be derived. It is pleasant to me to observe, Watson, that you have so far grasped this truth that in these little records of our cases which you have been good enough to draw up, and, I am bound to say, occasionally to embellish, you have given prominence not so much to the many causes *cetebres* and sensational trials in which I have figured but rather to those incidents which may have been trivial in themselves, but which have given room for those faculties of deduction and of logical synthesis which I have made my special province."

"And yet," said I, smiling, "I cannot quite hold myself *absolved* from the charge of sensationalism which has been urged against my records."

"You have erred, perhaps," he observed, taking up a glowing *cinder* with the tongs and lighting with it the long cherrywood pipe which was *wont* to replace his clay when he was in a disputatious rather than a meditative mood –"you have erred perhaps in attempting to put colour and life into each of your statements instead of confining yourself to the task of placing upon record that severe reasoning from cause to effect which is really the only notable feature about the thing."

"It seems to me that I have done you full justice in the matter," I remarked with some coldness, for I was repelled by the egotism which I had more than once observed to be a strong factor in my friend's singular character.

"No, it is not selfishness or *conceit*," said he, answering, as was his wont, my thoughts rather than my words. "If I claim full justice for my art, it is because it is an impersonal thing – a thing beyond myself. Crime is common. Logic is rare. Therefore it is upon the logic rather than upon the crime that you should dwell. You have degraded what should have been a course of lectures into a series of tales."

Cinder - *Partially or mostly burnt piece of coal*
Absolved - *To free from guilt or blame*
Embellish - *To beautify*
Célèbres – *Famous*
Wont – *In a habit of doing*

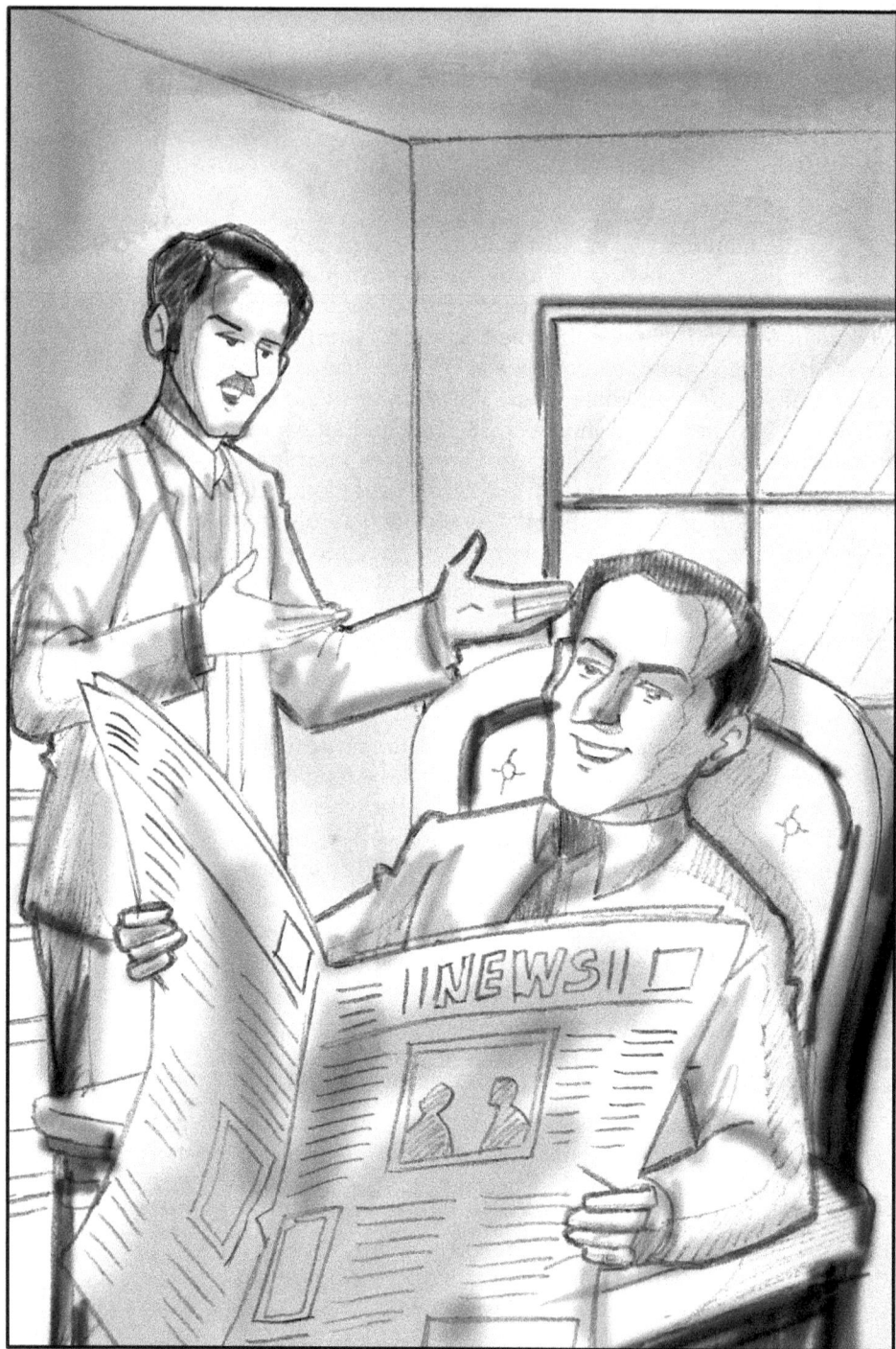

It was a cold morning of the early spring, and we sat after breakfast on either side of a cheery fire in the old room at Baker Street. A thick fog rolled down between the lines of *dun-colored* houses, and the opposing windows loomed like dark, shapeless blurs through the heavy yellow *wreaths*. Our gas was lit and shone on the white cloth and glimmer of china and metal, for the table had not been cleared yet. Sherlock Holmes had been silent all the morning, dipping continuously into the advertisement columns of a succession of papers until at last, having apparently given up his search, he had emerged in no very sweet temper to lecture me upon my literary shortcomings.

"At the same time," he remarked after a pause, during which he had sat puffing at his long pipe and gazing down into the fire, "you can hardly be open to a charge of sensation-alism, for out of these cases, which you have been so kind as to interest yourself in, a fair proportion do not treat of crime, in its legal sense, at all. The small matter in which I endeav-oured to help the King of Bohemia, the singular experience of Miss Mary Sutherland, the problem connected with the man with the twisted lip, and the incident of the noble bachelor, were all matters which are outside the *pale* of the law. But in avoiding the sensational, I fear that you may have bordered on the trivial."

"The end may have been so," I answered, "but the methods I hold to have been novel and of interest."

"Pshaw, my dear fellow, what do the public, the great unobservant public, who could hardly tell a weaver by his tooth or a compositor by his left thumb, care about the finer shades of analysis and deduction! But, indeed, if you are trivial. I cannot blame you, for the days of the great cases are past. Man, or at least criminal man, has lost all enterprise and originality. As to my own little practice, it seems to be degenerating into an agency for recovering lost lead pencils and giving advice to young ladies from boarding-schools. I think that I have touched bottom at last, however. This note I had this morning marks my zero-point, I fancy. Read it!" He tossed a crumpled letter across to me.

It was dated from Montague Place upon the preceding evening, and ran thus:

"DEAR MR. HOLMES,

Dun-coloured - *Dull-coloured*
Loomed - *Appear as a shadowy form*
Wreaths – *Garlands*
Pale – *An enclosed area*

I am very anxious to consult you as to whether, I should or should not accept a situation which has been offered to me as governess. I shall call at half-past ten tomorrow if I do not inconvenience you.

"Yours faithfully,
"VIOLET HUNTER."

"Do you know the young lady?" I asked.

"Not I."

"It is half-past ten now."

"Yes, and I have no doubt that is her ring."

"It may turn out to be of more interest than you think. You remember that the affair of the blue *carbuncle*, which appeared to be a mere whim at first, developed into a serious investigation. It may be so in this case, also."

"Well, let us hope so. But our doubts will very soon be solved, for here, unless I am much mistaken, is the person in question."

As he spoke the door opened and a young lady entered the room. She was plainly but neatly dressed, with a bright, quick face, freckled like a *plover's* egg, and with the brisk manner of a woman who has had her own way to make in the world.

"You will excuse my troubling you, I am sure," said she, as my companion rose to greet her, "but I have had a very strange experience, and as I have no parents or relations of any sort from whom I could ask advice, I thought that perhaps you would be kind enough to tell me what I should do."

"Pray take a seat, Miss Hunter. I shall be happy to do anything that I can to serve you."

I could see that Holmes was favourably impressed by the manner and speech of his new client. He looked her over in his searching fashion, and then composed himself, with his lids *drooping* and his finger-tips together, to listen to her story.

"I have been a governess for five years," said she, "in the family of Colonel Spence Munro, but two months ago, the colonel received an appointment at Halifax, in Nova Scotia, and took his children over to America with him, so that I found myself without a situation. I advertised, and I answered advertisements, but without success. At last the little money which I

Drooping -
Bending or hanging downwards
Carbuncle – *A bright and valuable gem*
Plover – *A bird*

had saved began to run short, and I was at my wits' end as to what I should do.

"There is a well-known agency for governesses in the West End called Westaway's, and there I used to call about once a week in order to see whether anything had turned up which might suit me. Westaway was the name of the founder of the business, but it is really managed by Miss Stoper. She sits in her own little office, and the ladies who are seeking employment wait in an *anteroom*, and are then shown in one by one, when she consults her ledgers and sees whether she has anything which would suit them.

"Well, when I called last week I was shown into the little office as usual, but I found that Miss Stoper was not alone. A *prodigiously* stout man with a very smiling face and a great heavy chin which rolled down in fold upon fold over his throat sat at her elbow with a pair of glasses on his nose, looking very earnestly at the ladies who entered. As I came in, he gave quite a jump in his chair and turned quickly to Miss Stoper.

"'That will do,' said he; 'I could not ask for anything better. Capital! capital!' He seemed quite enthusiastic and rubbed his hands together in the most *genial* fashion. He was such a comfortable-looking man that it was quite a pleasure to look at him.

"'You are looking for a situation, miss?' he asked.

"'Yes, sir.'

"'As governess?'

"'Yes, sir.'

"'And what salary do you ask?'

"'I had 4 pounds a month in my last place with Colonel Spence Munro.'

"'Oh, tut, tut! sweating – rank sweating!' he cried, throwing his fat hands out into the air like a man who is in a boiling passion. 'How could anyone offer so pitiful a sum to a lady with such attractions and accomplishments?'

"'My accomplishments, sir, may be less than you imagine,' said I. 'A little French, a little German, music, and drawing –'

"'Tut, tut!' he cried. 'This is all quite beside the question. The point is, have you or have you not the bearing and *deportment* of a lady? There it is in a nutshell. If you have not, you

Genial - *Friendly, cheerful*
Prodigiously - *Enormously*
Wits end - *To be very worried or upset*
Anteroom – *Waiting room*
Deportment – *Manner and behaviour*

are not fined for the *rearing* of a child who may some day try to play a considerable part in the history of the country. But if you have why, then, how could any gentleman ask you to *condescend* to accept anything under the three figures? Your salary with me, madam, would commence at 100 pounds a year.'

"You may imagine, Mr. Holmes, that to me, *destitute* as I was, such an offer seemed almost too good to be true. The gentleman, however, seeing perhaps the look of incredulity upon my face, opened a pocket-book and took out a note.

"'It is also my custom,' said he, smiling in the most pleasant fashion until his eyes were just two little shining slits amid the white creases of his face, 'to advance to my young ladies half their salary beforehand, so that they may meet any little expenses of their journey and their wardrobe.'

"It seemed to me that I had never met so fascinating and so thoughtful a man. As I was already in debt to my tradesmen, the advance was a great convenience, and yet there was something unnatural about the whole *transaction* which made me wish to know a little more before I quite committed myself.

"'May I ask where you live, sir?' said I.

"'Hampshire. Charming rural place. The Copper Beeches, five miles on the far side of Winchester. It is the most lovely country, my dear young lady, and the dearest old country-house.'

"'And my duties, sir? I should be glad to know what they would be.'

"'One child – one dear little *romper* just six years old. Oh, if you could see him killing cockroaches with a slipper! Smack! smack! smack! Three gone before you could wink!' He leaned back in his chair and laughed his eyes into his head again.

"I was a little startled at the nature of the child's amusement, but the father's laughter made me think that perhaps he was joking.

"'My sole duties, then,' I asked, 'are to take charge of a single child?'

"'No, no, not the sole, not the sole, my dear young lady,' he cried. 'Your duty would be, as I am sure your good sense would suggest, to obey any little commands my wife might

Propriety - *The state of being proper*
Transaction - *A business record*
Incredulity - *Disbelief*
Destitute - *Orphan*
Condescend - *To yield or to give assent to*
Rearing – *Nurture*
Romper – *A one-piece outer garment*

give, provided always that they were such commands as a lady might with *propriety* obey. You see no difficulty, heh?'

"'I should be happy to make myself useful.'

"'Quite so. In dress now, for example. We are *faddy* people, you know – faddy but kind-hearted. If you were asked to wear any dress which we might give you, you would not object to our little whim. Heh?'

"'No,' said I, considerably astonished at his words.

"'Or to sit here, or sit there, that would not be *offensive* to you?'

"'Oh, no.'

"'Or to cut your hair quite short before you come to us?'

"I could hardly believe my ears. As you may observe, Mr. Holmes, my hair is somewhat luxuriant, and of a rather peculiar tint of chestnut. It has been considered artistic. I could not dream of sacrificing it in this offhand fashion.

"'I am afraid that that is quite impossible,' said I. He had been watching me eagerly out of his small eyes, and I could see a shadow pass over his face as I spoke.

"'I am afraid that it is quite essential,' said he. 'It is a little fancy of my wife's, and ladies' fancies, you know, madam, ladies' fancies must be consulted. And so you won't cut your hair?'

"'No, sir, I really could not,' I answered firmly.

"'Ah, very well; then that quite settles the matter. It is a pity, because in other respects, you would really have done very nicely. In that case, Miss Stoper, I had best inspect a few more of your young ladies.'

"The manageress had sat all this while busy with her papers without a word to either of us, but she glanced at me now with so much annoyance upon her face that I could not help suspecting that she had lost a handsome commission through my refusal.

"'Do you desire your name to be kept upon the books?' she asked.

"'If you please, Miss Stoper.'

"'Well, really, it seems rather useless, since you refuse the most excellent offers in this fashion,' said she sharply. 'You can hardly expect us to exert ourselves to find another such opening for you. Good-day to you, Miss Hunter.' She struck a *gong* upon the table, and I was shown out by the page.

Offensive - *Annoying, Resentful, Displeasure*
Faddy – *A craze*
Gong – *Bell*

"Well, Mr. Holmes, when I got back to my lodgings and found little enough in the cupboard, and two or three bills upon the table. I began to ask myself whether I had not done a very foolish thing. After all, if these people had strange fads and expected obedience on the most extraordinary matters, they were at least ready to pay for their *eccentricity*. Very few governesses in England are getting 100 pounds a year. Besides, what use was my hair to me? Many people are improved by wearing it short and perhaps, I should be among the number. Next day, I was inclined to think that I had made a mistake, and by the day after I was sure of it. I had almost overcome my pride so far as to go back to the agency and inquire whether the place was still open when I received this letter from the gentleman himself. I have it here and I will read it to you:

"'The Copper Beeches, near Winchester.

"'DEAR MISS HUNTER,

"'Miss Stoper has very kindly given me your address, and I write from here to ask you whether you have reconsidered your decision. My wife is very anxious that you should come, for she has been much attracted by my description of you. We are willing to give 30 pounds a quarter, or 120 pounds a year, so as to *recompense* you for any little inconvenience which our *fads* may cause you. They are not very *exacting*, after all. My wife is fond of a particular shade of electric blue and would like you to wear such a dress indoors in the morning. You need not, however, go to the expense of purchasing one, as we have one belonging to my dear daughter Alice (now in Philadelphia), which would, I should think, fit you very well. Then, as to sitting here or there, or amusing yourself in any manner indicated, that need cause you no inconvenience. As regards your hair, it is no doubt a pity, especially as I could not help remarking its beauty during our short interview, but I am afraid that I must remain firm upon this point, and I only hope that the increased salary may recompense you for the loss. Your duties, as far as the child is concerned, are very light. Now do try to come, and I shall meet you with the dog-cart at Winchester. Let me know your train.

"'Yours faithfully,

"'JEPHRO RUCASTLE.'

Eccentricity - *Madness, Craziness*
Fads – *Enthusiasm about something for small periods*
Exacting – *Demanding*

"That is the letter which I have just received, Mr. Holmes, and my mind is made up that I will accept it. I thought, however, that before taking the final step, I should like to submit the whole matter to your consideration."

"Well, Miss Hunter, if your mind is made up, that settles the question," said Holmes, smiling.

"But you would not advise me to refuse?"

"I confess that it is not the situation which I should like to see a sister of mine apply for."

"What is the meaning of it all, Mr. Holmes?"

"Ah, I have no data. I cannot tell. Perhaps, you have yourself formed some opinion?"

"Well, there seems to me to be only one possible solution. Mr. Rucastle seemed to be a very kind, good-natured man. Is it not possible that his wife is a *lunatic*, that he desires to keep the matter quiet for fear she should be taken to an *asylum*, and that he humours her fancies in every way in order to prevent an outbreak?"

"That is a possible solution – in fact, as matters stand, it is the most probable one. But in any case, it does not seem to be a nice household for a young lady."

"But the money, Mr. Holmes, the money!"

"Well, yes, of course, the pay is good – too good. That is what makes me uneasy. Why should they give you 120 pounds a year, when they could have their pick for 40 pounds? There must be some strong reason behind."

"I thought that if I told you the circumstances, you would understand afterwards if I wanted your help. I should feel so much stronger if I felt that you were at the back of me." "Oh, you may carry that feeling away with you. I assure you that your little problem promises to be the most interesting which has come my way for some months. There is something distinctly novel about some of the features. If you should find yourself in doubt or in danger –"

"Danger! What danger do you foresee?"

Holmes shook his head *gravely*. "It would cease to be a danger if we could define it," said he. "But at any time, day or night, a telegram would bring me down to your help."

"That is enough." She rose *briskly* from her chair with the anxiety all swept from her face. "I shall go down to Hampshire

Briskly - *Quickly, Actively*
Gravely - *Seriously*
Lunatic – *Crazy person*
Asylum – *Insane Shelter for special people*

quite easy in my mind now. I shall write to Mr. Rucastle at once, sacrifice my poor hair tonight, and start for Winchester tomorrow." With a few grateful words to Holmes, she bade us both goodnight and bustled off upon her way.

"At least," said I as we heard her quick, firm steps descending the stairs, "she seems to be a young lady who is very well able to take care of herself."

"And she would need to be," said Holmes gravely. "I am much mistaken if we do not hear from her before many days are past."

It was not very long before my friend's prediction was fulfilled. A fortnight went by, during which I frequently found my thoughts turning in her direction and wondering what strange side-alley of human experience this lonely woman had **strayed** into. The unusual salary, the curious conditions, the light duties, all pointed to something abnormal, though whether a fad or a plot, or whether the man were a **philanthropist** or a villain, it was quite beyond my powers to determine. As to Holmes, I observed that he sat frequently for half an hour on end, with knitted brows and an **abstracted** air, but he swept the matter away with a wave of his hand when I mentioned it. "Data! data! data!" he cried impatiently. "I can't make bricks without clay." And yet he would always wind up by muttering that no sister of his should ever have accepted such a situation.

The telegram which we eventually received came late one night just as I was thinking of turning in and Holmes was settling down to one of those all-night chemical researches which he frequently indulged in, when I would leave him stooping over a **retort** and a test-tube at night and find him in the same position when I came down to breakfast in the morning. He opened the yellow envelope, and then, glancing at the message, threw it across to me.

"Just look up the trains in Bradshaw," said he, and turned back to his chemical studies. The summons was a brief and urgent one:

"Please be at the Black Swan Hotel at Winchester at midday tomorrow," it said."Do come! I am at my wit's end. HUNTER."

"Will you come with me?" asked Holmes, glancing up.

"I should wish to."

"Just look it up, then."

Abstracted - *Lost in thoughts*
Strayed - *To deviate from the direct course*
Philanthropist – *Generous donor*
Retort – *Angry reply*

"There is a train at half-past nine," said I, glancing over my Bradshaw. "It is due at Winchester at 11:30."

"That will do very nicely. Then perhaps, I had better postpone my analysis of the acetones, as we may need to be at our best in the morning."

By eleven o'clock, the next day we were well upon our way to the old English capital. Holmes had been buried in the morning papers all the way down, but after we had passed the Hampshire border, he threw them down and began to admire the scenery. It was an ideal spring day, a light blue sky, *flecked* with little *fleecy* white clouds drifting across from west to east. The sun was shining very brightly, and yet there was an *exhilarating* nip in the air, which set an edge to a man's energy. All over the countryside, away to the rolling hills around Aldershot, the little red and grey roofs of the farm-steadings peeped out from amid the light green of the new foliage.

"Are they not fresh and beautiful?" I cried with all the enthusiasm of a man fresh from the fogs of Baker Street.

But Holmes shook his head gravely.

"Do you know, Watson," said he, "that it is one of the curses of a mind with a turn like mine that I must look at everything with reference to my own special subject. You look at these scattered houses, and you are impressed by their beauty. I look at them, and the only thought which comes to me is a feeling of their isolation and of the *impunity* with which crime may be committed there."

"Good heavens!" I cried. "Who would associate crime with these dear old *homesteads*?"

"They always fill me with a certain horror. It is my belief, Watson, founded upon my experience, that the lowest and *vilest* alleys in London do not present a more dreadful record of sin than does the smiling and beautiful countryside."

"You horrify me!"

"But the reason is very obvious. The pressure of public opinion can do in the town what the law cannot accomplish. There is no lane so vile that the scream of a tortured child, or the thud of a drunkard's blow, does not beget sympathy and indignation among the neighbours, and then the whole machinery of justice is ever so close that a word of complaint

Vilest - *Highly offensive*

Fleecy - *Resembling a wool*

Impunity - *Exemption from punishment*

Flecked – *Marked*

Homesteads – *Houses*

can set it going, and there is but a step between the crime and the dock. But look at these lonely houses, each in its own fields, filled for the most part with poor ignorant folk who know little of the law. Think of the deeds of hellish cruelty, the hidden wickedness which may go on, year in, year out, in such places, and none the wiser. Had this lady who appeals to us for help gone to live in Winchester, I should never have had a fear for her. It is the five miles of country which makes the danger. Still, it is clear that she is not personally threatened."

"No. If she can come to Winchester to meet us, she can get away."

"Quite so. She has her freedom."

"What can be the matter, then? Can you suggest no explanation?"

"I have devised seven separate explanations, each of which would cover the facts as far as we know them. But which of these is correct can only be determined by the fresh information which we shall no doubt find waiting for us. Well, there is the tower of the cathedral, and we shall soon learn all that Miss Hunter has to tell."

The Black Swan is an inn of *repute* in the High Street, at no distance from the station, and there we found the young lady waiting for us. She had engaged a sitting room, and our lunch awaited us upon the table.

"I am so delighted that you have come," she said *earnestly*. "It is so very kind of you both; but indeed I do not know what I should do. Your advice will be altogether invaluable to me."

"Pray tell us what has happened to you."

"I will do so, and I must be quick, for I have promised Mr. Rucastle to be back before three. I got his leave to come into town this morning, though he little knew for what purpose."

"Let us have everything in its due order." Holmes thrust his long thin legs out towards the fire and composed himself to listen.

"In the first place, I may say that I have met, on the whole, with no actual ill-treatment from Mr. and Mrs. Rucastle. It is only fair to them to say that. But I cannot understand them, and I am not easy in my mind about them."

"What can you not understand?"

Repute – *Reputation, Name in the society*
Earnestly – *Sincerely*

Greatest Adventure Stories of Sherlock Holmes - 2

"Their reasons for their conduct. But you shall have it all just as it occurred. When I came down, Mr. Rucastle met me here and drove me in his dog-cart to the Copper Beeches. It is, as he said, beautifully situated, but it is not beautiful in itself, for it is a large square block of a house, whitewashed, but all stained and streaked with damp and bad weather. There are grounds around it, woods on three sides, and on the fourth, a field which slopes down to the Southampton highroad, which curves past about a hundred yards from the front door. This ground in front belongs to the house, but the woods all around are part of Lord Southerton's preserves. A clump of copper beeches immediately in front of the hall door has given its name to the place.

"I was driven over by my employer, who was as *amiable* as ever, and was introduced by him that evening to his wife and the child. There was no truth, Mr. Holmes, in the conjecture which seemed to us to be probable in your rooms at Baker Street. Mrs. Rucastle is not mad. I found her to be a silent, pale-faced woman, much younger than her husband, not more than thirty, I should think, while he can hardly be less than forty-five. From their conversation, I have gathered that they have been married about seven years, that he was a widower, and that his only child by the first wife was the daughter who has gone to Philadelphia. Mr. Rucastle told me in private that the reason why she had left them was that she had an unreasoning *aversion* to her stepmother. As the daughter could not have been less than twenty, I can quite imagine that her position must have been uncomfortable with her father's young wife.

"Mrs. Rucastle seemed to me to be *colorless* in mind as well as in features. She impressed me neither favourably nor the reverse. She was a *nonentity*. It was easy to see that she was passionately devoted both to her husband and to her little son. Her light grey eyes wandered continually from one to the other, noting every little wants and *forestalling* it if possible. He was kind to her also in his bluff, *boisterous* fashion, and on the whole, they seemed to be a happy couple. And yet she, had some secret sorrow, this woman. She would often be lost in deep thought, with the saddest look upon her face. More than once, I have surprised her in tears. I have thought sometimes that it was the *disposition* of her child which weighed upon her mind, for I have never met so utterly

Aversion - *A strong belief of dislike*
Amiable - *Agreeable, friendly*
Nonentity – *Nobody*
Forestalling – *Preventing or putting something off*

spoiled and so ill-natured a little creature. He is small for his age, with a head which is quite disproportionately large. His whole life appears to be spent in an alternation between savage fits of passion and gloomy intervals of sulking. Giving pain to any creature weaker than himself seems to be his one idea of amusement, and he shows quite remarkable talent in planning the capture of mice, little birds, and insects. But I would rather not talk about the creature, Mr. Holmes, and, indeed, he has little to do with my story."

"I am glad of all details," remarked my friend, "whether they seem to you to be relevant or not."

"I shall try not to miss anything of importance. The one unpleasant thing about the house, which struck me at once, was the appearance and conduct of the servants. There are only two, a man and his wife. Toller, for that is his name, is a rough, **uncouth** man, with grizzled hair and whiskers, and a **perpetual** smell of drink. Twice since I have been with them, he has been quite drunk, and yet Mr. Rucastle seemed to take no notice of it. His wife is a very tall and strong woman with a sour face, as silent as Mrs. Rucastle and much less amiable. They are a most unpleasant couple, but fortunately, I spend most of my time in the nursery and my own room, which are next to each other in one corner of the building.

"For two days after my arrival at the Copper Beeches, my life was very quiet; on the third, Mrs. Rucastle came down just after breakfast and whispered something to her husband. "'Oh, yes,' said he, turning to me, 'we are very much obliged to you, Miss Hunter, for falling in with our whims so far as to cut your hair. I assure you that it has not **detracted** in the tiniest **iota** from your appearance. We shall now see how the electric-blue dress will become you. You will find it laid out upon the bed in your room, and if you would be so good as to put it on, we should both be extremely obliged.'

"The dress which I found waiting for me was of a peculiar shade of blue. It was of excellent material, a sort of beige, but it bore unmistakable signs of having been worn before. It could not have been a better fit if I had been measured for it. Both Mr. and Mrs. Rucastle expressed a delight at the look of it, which seemed quite exaggerated in its **vehemence**. They were waiting for me in the drawing room, which is a very large room, stretching along the entire front of the house, with

Vehemence - *Fury*
Detracted - *Distracted, To draw away or divert*
Iota - *A very small quantity*
Uncouth – *Uncivilized*
Perpetual – *Continuous*

three long windows reaching down to the floor. A chair had been placed close to the central window, with its back turned towards it. In this I was asked to sit, and then Mr. Rucastle, walking up and down on the other side of the room, began to tell me a series of the funniest stories that I have ever listened to. You cannot imagine how comical he was, and I laughed until I was quite weary. Mrs. Rucastle, however, who has evidently no sense of humour, never so much as smiled, but sat with her hands in her lap, and a sad, anxious look upon her face. After an hour or so, Mr. Rucastle suddenly remarked that it was time to commence the duties of the day, and that I might change my dress and go to little Edward in the nursery.

"Two days later, this same performance was gone through under exactly similar circumstances. Again I changed my dress, again I sat in the window, and again I laughed very heartily at the funny stories of which my employer had an immense *repertoire*, and which he told *inimitably*. Then he handed me a yellow-backed novel, and moving my chair a little sideways, that my own shadow might not fall upon the page, he begged me to read aloud to him. I read for about ten minutes, beginning in the heart of a chapter, and then suddenly, in the middle of a sentence, he ordered me to cease and to change my dress.

"You can easily imagine, Mr. Holmes, how curious I became as to what the meaning of this extraordinary performance could possibly be. They were always very careful, I observed, to turn my face away from the window, so that I became consumed with the desire to see what was going on behind my back. At first it seemed to be impossible, but I soon devised a means. My hand-mirror had been broken, so a happy thought seized me, and I concealed a piece of the glass in my handkerchief. On the next occasion, in the midst of my laughter, I put my handkerchief up to my eyes, and was able with a little management to see all that there was behind me. I confess that I was disappointed. There was nothing. At least that was my first impression. At the second glance, however, I perceived that there was a man standing in the Southampton Road, a small bearded man in a grey suit, who seemed to be looking in my direction. The road is an important highway, and there are usually people there. This man, however, was leaning against the railings which bordered our field and was

Impertinent -
Irrelevant
Repertoire –
Collection
Inimitably –
Exclusively

looking earnestly up. I lowered my handkerchief and glanced at Mrs. Rucastle to find her eyes fixed upon me with a most searching gaze. She said nothing, but I am convinced that she had divined that I had a mirror in my hand and had seen what was behind me. She rose at once. "'Jephro,' said she, 'there is an impertinent fellow upon the road there who stares up at Miss Hunter.'

"'No friend of yours, Miss Hunter?' he asked.

"'No, I know no one in these parts.'

"'Dear me! How very impertinent! Kindly turn around and motion to him to go away.'

"'Surely it would be better to take no notice.'

"'No, no, we should have him loitering here always. Kindly turn around and wave him away like that.'

"I did as I was told, and at the same instant, Mrs. Rucastle drew down the blind. That was a week ago, and from that time I have not sat again in the window, nor have I worn the blue dress, nor seen the man in the road."

"Pray continue," said Holmes. "Your narrative promises to be a most interesting one."

"You will find it rather disconnected, I fear, and there may prove to be little relation between the different incidents of which I speak. On the very first day that I was at the Copper Beeches, Mr. Rucastle took me to a small outhouse which stands near the kitchen door. As we approached it, I heard the sharp rattling of a chain, and the sound as of a large animal moving about.

"'Look in here!' said Mr. Rucastle, showing me a slit between two planks. 'Is he not a beauty?' "I looked through and was conscious of two glowing eyes, and of a vague figure huddled up in the darkness.

"'Don't be frightened,' said my employer, laughing at the start which I had given. 'It's only Carlo, my **mastiff**. I call him mine, but really old Toller, my groom, is the only man who can do anything with him. We feed him once a day, and not too much then, so that he is always as keen as mustard. Toller lets him loose every night, and God help the trespasser whom he lays his fangs upon. For goodness' sake don't you ever on any pretext set your foot over the threshold at night, for it's as much as your life is worth.'

Mastiff – *A dog of a strong breed*
Rapt – *Captivated*

Greatest Adventure Stories of Sherlock Holmes - 2

"The warning was no idle one, for two nights later, I happened to look out of my bedroom window about two o'clock in the morning. It was a beautiful moonlit night, and the lawn in front of the house was silvered over and almost as bright as day. I was standing, *rapt* in the peaceful beauty of the scene, when I was aware that something was moving under the shadow of the copper beeches. As it emerged into the moonshine, I saw what it was. It was a giant dog, as large as a calf, *tawny tinted,* with hanging jowl, black muzzle, and huge projecting bones. It walked slowly across the lawn and vanished into the shadow upon the other side. That dreadful sentinel sent a chill to my heart which I do not think that any burglar could have done.

"And now I have a very strange experience to tell you. I had, as you know, cut off my hair in London, and I had placed it in a great coil at the bottom of my trunk. One evening, after the child was in bed, I began to amuse myself by examining the furniture of my room and by rearranging my own little things. There was an old chest of drawers in the room, the two upper ones empty and open, the lower one locked. I had filled the first two with my linen, and as I had still much to pack away, I was naturally annoyed at not having the use of the third drawer. It struck me that it might have been fastened by a mere oversight, so I took out my bunch of keys and tried to open it. The very first key fitted to perfection, and I drew the drawer open. There was only one thing in it, but I am sure that you would never guess what it was. It was my coil of hair.

"I took it up and examined it. It was of the same peculiar tint, and the same thickness. But then the impossibility of the thing *obtruded* itself upon me. How could my hair have been locked in the drawer? With trembling hands I undid my trunk, turned out the contents, and drew from the bottom my own hair. I laid the two tresses together, and I assure you that they were identical. Was it not extraordinary? Puzzle as I would, I could make nothing at all of what it meant. I returned the strange hair to the drawer, and I said nothing of the matter to the Rucastles as I felt that I had put myself in the wrong by opening a drawer which they had locked.

"I am naturally observant, as you may have remarked, Mr. Holmes, and I soon had a pretty good plan of the whole

Jowle - *Lower jaw*
Jovial - *Cheerful*
Crinkled - *Wrinkled*
Muzzle - *Mouth of a barrel*
Linen – *A type of cloth*
Obtruded – *Thrust out or between something*

house in my head. There was one wing, however, which appeared not to be inhabited at all. A door which faced that which led into the quarters of the Tollers opened into this suite, but it was invariably locked. One day, however, as I ascended the stair, I met Mr. Rucastle coming out through this door, his keys in his hand, and a look on his face which made him a very different person to the round, jovial man to whom I was accustomed. His cheeks were red, his brow was all *crinkled* with anger, and the veins stood out at his temples with passion. He locked the door and hurried past me without a word or a look.

"This aroused my curiosity, so when I went out for a walk in the grounds with my charge, I strolled around to the side from which I could see the windows of this part of the house. There were four of them in a row, three of which were simply dirty, while the fourth was *shuttered* up. They were evidently all *deserted*. As I strolled up and down, *glancing* at them occasionally, Mr. Rucastle came out to me, looking as merry and jovial as ever.

"'Ah!' said he, 'you must not think me rude if I passed you without a word, my dear young lady. I was *preoccupied* with business matters.'

"I assured him that I was not offended. 'By the way,' said I, 'you seem to have quite a suite of spare rooms up there, and one of them has the shutters up.'

"He looked surprised and, as it seemed to me, a little *startled* at my remark.

"'Photography is one of my hobbies,' said he. 'I have made my dark room up there. But, dear me! What an observant young lady we have come upon. Who would have believed it? Who would have ever believed it?' He spoke in a jesting tone, but there was no jest in his eyes as he looked at me. I read suspicion there and annoyance, but no jest.

"Well, Mr. Holmes, from the moment that I understood that there was something about that suite of rooms which I was not to know, I was all on fire to go over them. It was not mere curiosity, though I have my share of that. It was more a feeling of duty – a feeling that some good might come from my penetrating to this place. They talk of woman's instinct; perhaps it was woman's instinct which gave me that feeling.

Shuttered – *Shut down*
Forbidden - *Prohibited*
Startled - *Very surprised*
Preoccupied - *Busy*
Glancing - *Quick look*
Deserted - *Forsakened, Abandoned*

At any rate, it was there, and I was keenly on the lookout for any chance to pass the *forbidden* door.

"It was only yesterday that the chance came. I may tell you that, besides Mr. Rucastle, both Toller and his wife find something to do in these deserted rooms, and I once saw him carrying a large black linen bag with him through the door. Recently, he has been drinking hard, and yesterday evening, he was very drunk; and when I came upstairs, there was the key in the door. I have no doubt at all that he had left it there. Mr. and Mrs. Rucastle were both downstairs, and the child was with them, so that I had an admirable opportunity. I turned the key gently in the lock, opened the door, and slipped through.

"There was a little passage in front of me, unpapered and uncarpeted, which turned at a right angle at the farther end. Round this corner were three doors in a line, the first and third of which were open. They each led into an empty room, dusty and cheerless, with two windows in the one and one in the other, so thick with dirt that the evening light glimmered dimly through them. The centre door was closed, and across the outside of it had been fastened one of the broad bars of an iron bed, padlocked at one end to a ring in the wall, and fastened at the other with stout cord. The door itself was locked as well, and the key was not there. This *barricaded* door corresponded clearly with the shuttered window outside, and yet I could see by the glimmer from beneath it that the room was not in darkness. Evidently, there was a skylight which let in light from above. As I stood in the passage gazing at the sinister door and wondering what secret it might veil, I suddenly heard the sound of steps within the room and saw a shadow pass backward and forward against the little slit of dim light which shone out from under the door. A mad, unreasoning terror rose up in me at the sight, Mr. Holmes. My *overstrung* nerves failed me suddenly, and I turned and ran – ran as though some dreadful hand were behind me clutching at the skirt of my dress. I rushed down the passage, through the door, and straight into the arms of Mr. Rucastle, who was waiting outside.

"'So,' said he, smiling, 'it was you, then. I thought that it must be when I saw the door open.' "'Oh, I am so frightened!' I *panted*.

Barricaded - *Fortified*
Panted - *Breathed*
Caressing - *Expressing affection*
Overstrung – *Extremely nervous*
Coaxing – *Persuading*

"'My dear young lady! my dear young lady!' – you cannot think how caressing and soothing his manner was – 'and what has frightened you, my dear young lady?'

"But his voice was just a little too **coaxing**. He overdid it. I was keenly on my guard against him.

"'I was foolish enough to go into the empty wing,' I answered. 'But it is so lonely and *eerie* in this dim light that I was frightened and ran out again. Oh, it is so dreadfully still in there!'

"'Only that?' said he, looking at me keenly.

"'Why, what did you think?' I asked.

"'Why do you think that I lock this door?'

"'I am sure that I do not know.'

"'It is to keep people out who have no business there. Do you see?' He was still smiling in the most amiable manner.

"'I am sure if I had known –'

"'Well, then, you know now. And if you ever put your foot over that threshold again' – here in an instant the smile hardened into a grin of rage, and he glared down at me with the face of a demon – 'I'll throw you to the mastiff.'

"I was so terrified that I do not know what I did. I suppose that I must have rushed past him into my room. I remember nothing until I found myself lying on my bed trembling all over. Then I thought of you, Mr. Holmes. I could not live there longer without some advice. I was frightened of the house, of the man, of the woman, of the servants, even of the child. They were all horrible to me. If I could only bring you down all would be well. Of course, I might have fled from the house, but my curiosity was almost as strong as my fears. My mind was soon made up. I would send you a wire. I put on my hat and cloak, went down to the office, which is about half a mile from the house, and then returned, feeling very much easier. A horrible doubt came into my mind as I approached the door lest the dog might be loose, but I remembered that Toller had drunk himself into a state of insensibility that evening, and I knew that he was the only one in the household who had any influence with the savage creature, or who would venture to set him free. I slipped in safety and lay awake half the night in my joy at the thought of seeing you. I had no difficulty in getting leave to come into

Threshold - *The entrance or sill of a doorway*
Spellbound – *Fascinated*
Profound – *Deep*

Winchester this morning, but I must be back before three o'clock, for Mr. and Mrs. Rucastle are going on a visit, and will be away all the evening, so that I must look after the child. Now I have told you all my adventures, Mr. Holmes, and I should be very glad if you could tell me what it all means, and, above all, what I should do."

Holmes and I had listened **spellbound** to this extraordinary story. My friend rose now and paced up and down the room, his hands in his pockets, and an expression of the most **profound** gravity upon his face.

"Is Toller still drunk?" he asked.

"Yes. I heard his wife tell Mrs. Rucastle that she could do nothing with him."

"That is well. And the Rucastles go out tonight?"

"Yes."

"Is there a cellar with a good strong lock?"

"Yes, the wine-cellar."

"You seem to me to have acted all through this matter like a very brave and sensible girl, Miss Hunter. Do you think that you could perform one more feat? I should not ask it of you if I did not think you a quite exceptional woman."

"I will try. What is it?"

"We shall be at the Copper Beeches by seven o'clock, my friend and I. The Rucastles will be gone by that time, and Toller will, we hope, be incapable. There only remains Mrs. Toller, who might give the alarm. If you could send her into the cellar on some **errand**, and then turn the key upon her, you would facilitate matters immensely."

"I will do it."

"Excellent! We shall then look thoroughly into the affair. Of course, there is only one **feasible** explanation. You have been brought there to **personate** someone, and the real person is imprisoned in this chamber. That is obvious. As to who this prisoner is, I have no doubt that it is the daughter, Miss Alice Rucastle, if I remember right, who was said to have gone to America. You were chosen, doubtless, as resembling her in height, figure, and the colour of your hair. Hers had been cut off, very possibly in some illness through which she has passed, and so, of course, yours had to be sacrificed also.

Tresses - *Long locks or curls of hair*
Personate - *To act or portray*
Feasible - *Suitable*
Errand – *Short trip for some work*
Disposition – *Nature and character*

By a curious chance, you came upon her *tresses*. The man in the road was undoubtedly some friend of hers – possibly her fiance – and no doubt, as you wore the girl's dress and were so like her, he was convinced from your laughter, whenever he saw you, and afterwards from your gesture, that Miss Rucastle was perfectly happy, and that she no longer desired his attentions. The dog is let loose at night to prevent him from endeavouring to communicate with her. So much is fairly clear. The most serious point in the case is the *disposition* of the child."

"What on earth has that to do with it?" I ejaculated.

"My dear Watson, you as a medical man are continually gaining light as to the tendencies of a child by the study of the parents. Don't you see that the converse is equally valid. I have frequently gained my first real insight into the character of parents by studying their children. This child's disposition is abnormally cruel, merely for cruelty's sake, and whether he derives this from his smiling father, as I should suspect, or from his mother, it bodes evil for the poor girl who is in their power."

"I am sure that you are right, Mr. Holmes," cried our client. "A thousand things come back to me which make me certain that you have hit it. Oh, let us lose not an instant in bringing help to this poor creature."

"We must be *circumspect*, for we are dealing with a very cunning man. We can do nothing until seven o'clock. At that hour, we shall be with you, and it will not be long before we solve the mystery."

We were as good as our word, for it was just seven when we reached the Copper Beeches, having put up our trap at a wayside public-house. The group of trees, with their dark leaves shining like *burnished* metal in the light of the setting sun, were sufficient to mark the house even had Miss Hunter not been standing smiling on the doorstep.

"Have you managed it?" asked Holmes.

A loud thudding noise came from somewhere downstairs. "That is Mrs. Toller in the cellar," said she. "Her husband lies snoring on the kitchen rug. Here are his keys, which are the duplicates of Mr. Rucastle's."

Rickety - *Shaky, likely to fall or collapse*
Transverse - *Cross*
Palletbed - *A mattress or bed of straw*
Circumspect – *Cautious*
Burnished – *Glossy*

"You have done well indeed!" cried Holmes with enthusiasm. "Now lead the way, and we shall soon see the end of this black business."

We passed up the stair, unlocked the door, followed on down a passage, and found ourselves in front of the barricade which Miss Hunter had described. Holmes cut the cord and removed the *transverse* bar. Then he tried the various keys in the lock, but without success. No sound came from within, and at the silence, Holmes's face clouded over.

"I trust that we are not too late," said he. "I think, Miss Hunter, that we had better go in without you. Now, Watson, put your shoulder to it, and we shall see whether we cannot make our way in."

It was an old *rickety* door and gave at once before our united strength. Together we rushed into the room. It was empty. There was no furniture save a little *pallet bed,* a small table, and a basketful of linen. The skylight above was open, and the prisoner gone.

"There has been some villainy here," said Holmes; "this beauty has guessed Miss Hunter's intentions and has carried his victim off."

"But how?"

"Through the skylight. We shall soon see how he managed it." He swung himself up onto the roof. "Ah, yes," he cried, "here's the end of a long light ladder against the *eaves*. That is how he did it."

"But it is impossible," said Miss Hunter; "the ladder was not there when the Rucastles went away."

"He has come back and done it. I tell you that he is a clever and dangerous man. I should not be very much surprised if this were he whose step I hear now upon the stair. I think, Watson, that it would be as well for you to have your pistol ready."

The words were hardly out of his mouth before a man appeared at the door of the room, a very fat and *burly* man, with a heavy stick in his hand. Miss Hunter screamed and shrunk against the wall at the sight of him, but Sherlock Holmes sprang forward and confronted him. "You villain!" said he, "where's your daughter?"

Burly - *Sturdy*
Eaves – *Attic*
Famished – *Hungry*

The fat man cast his eyes around, and then up at the open skylight.

"It is for me to ask you that," he shrieked, "you thieves! Spies and thieves! I have caught you, have I? You are in my power. I'll serve you!" He turned and clattered down the stairs as hard as he could go.

"He's gone for the dog!" cried Miss Hunter.

"I have my revolver," said I.

"Better close the front door," cried Holmes, and we all rushed down the stairs together. We had hardly reached the hall when we heard the baying of a hound, and then a scream of agony, with a horrible worrying sound which it was dreadful to listen to. An elderly man with a red face and shaking limbs came staggering out at a side door.

"My God!" he cried. "Someone has loosed the dog. It's not been fed for two days. Quick, quick, or it'll be too late!"

Holmes and I rushed out and around the angle of the house, with Toller hurrying behind us. There was the huge *famished* brute, its black *muzzle* buried in Rucastle's throat, while he *writhed* and screamed upon the ground. Running up, I blew its brains out, and it fell over with its keen white teeth still meeting in the great *creases* of his neck. With much labour, we separated them and carried him, living but horribly *mangled*, into the house. We laid him upon the drawing room sofa, and having dispatched the sobered Toller to bear the news to his wife, I did what I could to relieve his pain. We were all assembled around him when the door opened, and a tall, *gaunt* woman entered the room.

"Mrs. Toller!" cried Miss Hunter.

"Yes, miss. Mr. Rucastle let me out when he came back before he went up to you. Ah, miss, it is a pity you didn't let me know what you were planning, for I would have told you that your pains were wasted."

"Ha!" said Holmes, looking keenly at her. "It is clear that Mrs. Toller knows more about this matter than anyone else."

"Yes, sir, I do, and I am ready enough to tell what I know."

"Then, pray, sit down, and let us hear it for there are several points on which I must confess that I am still in the dark."

Gaunt - *Very thin and bony*
Writhed – *Twisted and contorted*
Slighted – *Affronted*

"I will soon make it clear to you," said she; "and I'd have done so before now if I could ha' got out from the cellar. If there's police-court business over this, you'll remember that I was the one that stood your friend, and that I was Miss Alice's friend too.

"She was never happy at home, Miss Alice wasn't, from the time that her father married again. She was **slighted** like and had no say in anything, but it never really became bad for her until after she met Mr. Fowler at a friend's house. As well as I could learn, Miss Alice had rights of her own by will, but she was so quiet and patient, she was, that she never said a word about them but just left everything in Mr. Rucastle's hands. He knew he was safe with her; but when there was a chance of a husband coming forward, who would ask for all that the law would give him, then her father thought it time to put a stop on it. He wanted her to sign a paper, so that whether she married or not, he could use her money. When she wouldn't do it, he kept on worrying her until she got brain-fever, and for six weeks was at death's door. Then she got better at last, all worn to a shadow, and with her beautiful hair cut off; but that didn't make no change in her young man, and he stuck to her as true as man could be."

"Ah," said Holmes, "I think that what you have been good enough to tell us makes the matter fairly clear, and that I can deduce all that remains. Mr. Rucastle then, I presume, took to this system of imprisonment?"

"Yes, sir."

"And brought Miss Hunter down from London in order to get rid of the disagreeable persistence of Mr. Fowler."

"That was it, sir."

"But Mr. Fowler being a **persevering** man, as a good seaman should be, the house, and having met you succeeded by certain arguments, metallic or otherwise, in convincing you that your interests were the same as his."

"Mr. Fowler was a very kind-spoken, free-handed gentleman," said Mrs. Toller **serenely**.

"And in this way, he managed that your good man should have no want of drink, and that a ladder should be ready at the moment when your master had gone out."

"You have it, sir, just as it happened."

Deduce - *To derive or infer*

Persevering - *Showing relentless steadfastness*

Serenely - *Calmly*

Blockaded – *Blocked*

Locus standi – *Right to be heard in court*

"I am sure we owe you an apology, Mrs. Toller," said Holmes, "for you have certainly cleared up everything which puzzled us. And here comes the country surgeon and Mrs. Rucastle, so I think. Watson, that we had best escort Miss Hunter back to Winchester, as it seems to me that our *locus standi* now is rather a questionable one."

And thus was solved the mystery of the sinister house with the copper beeches in front of the door. Mr. Rucastle survived, but was always a broken man, kept alive solely through the care of his devoted wife. They still live with their old servants, who probably know so much of Rucastle's past life that he finds it difficult to part from them. Mr. Fowler and Miss Rucastle were married, by special license, in Southampton the day after their flight, and he is now the holder of a government appointment in the island of Mauritius. As to Miss Violet Hunter, my friend Holmes, rather to my disappointment, *manifested* no further interest in her when once she had ceased to be the centre of one of his problems, and she is now the head of a private school at Walsall, where I believe that she has met with considerable success.

Locus Standi - *Right to be heard in court*
Manifested – *Evident, Obvious, Apparent*

Food For Thought

If Miss Hunter had not been asked to cut her hair short to procure the job, how would have Holmes been able to solve this mysterious case?

An Understanding

Q. 1. Why was Miss Violet Hunter in a dilemma to accept a situation which had been offered to her as a governess?
Ans. _____
_____
_____
_____
_____

Q. 2. Why did Mr. Rucastle offer such a high and attractive salary of 120 pounds a year to Miss Violet Hunter?
Ans. _____
_____
_____
_____
_____

Q. 3. How did Sherlock Holmes's prediction come true? What was his prediction regarding Miss Hunter's new and strange job at Winchester?
Ans. _____
_____
_____
_____
_____

Q. 4. "Jephro." said she, "There is an impertinent fellow upon the road there, who stares up at Miss Hunter." Who said the above dialogue to whom? Why did the narrator utter the above words?
Ans. _____
_____
_____
_____
_____

The Adventure of the Blue Carbuncle

~Arthur Conan Doyle

I had called upon my friend Sherlock Holmes upon the second morning after Christmas, with the intention of wishing him the compliments of the season. He was lounging upon the sofa in a purple dressing-gown, a pipe-rack within his reach upon the right, and a pile of crumpled morning papers, evidently newly studied, near at hand. Beside the couch, was a wooden chair, and on the angle of the back hung a very seedy and disreputable hard-felt hat, much the worse for wear, and cracked in several places. A lens and a *forceps* lying upon the seat of the chair suggested that the hat had been suspended in this manner for the purpose of examination.

"You are engaged," said I; "perhaps I interrupt you."

"Not at all. I am glad to have a friend with whom I can discuss my results. The matter is a perfectly *trivial* one" – he jerked his thumb in the direction of the old hat – "but there are points in connection with it which are not entirely devoid of interest and even of instruction." I seated myself in his armchair and warmed my hands before his *crackling* fire, for a sharp frost had set in, and the windows were thick with the ice crystals. "I suppose," I remarked, "that, homely as it looks, this thing has some deadly story linked on to it – that it is the clue which will guide you in the solution of some mystery and the punishment of some crime."

"No, no. No crime," said Sherlock Holmes, laughing. "Only one of those whimsical little incidents which will happen when you have four million human beings all jostling each other within the space of a few square miles. Amid the action and reaction of so dense a swarm of humanity, every possible combination of events may be expected to take place, and many a little problem will be presented which may be striking and *bizarre* without being criminal. We have already had experience of such."

"So much so," I remarked, "that of the last six cases which I have added to my notes, three have been entirely free of any legal crime."

Devoid - *To deplete or strip of*
Trivial - *Unimportant*
Forcep - *A surgical instrument*
Crackling – *Making sharp snapping noise*
Bizarre – *Strange*

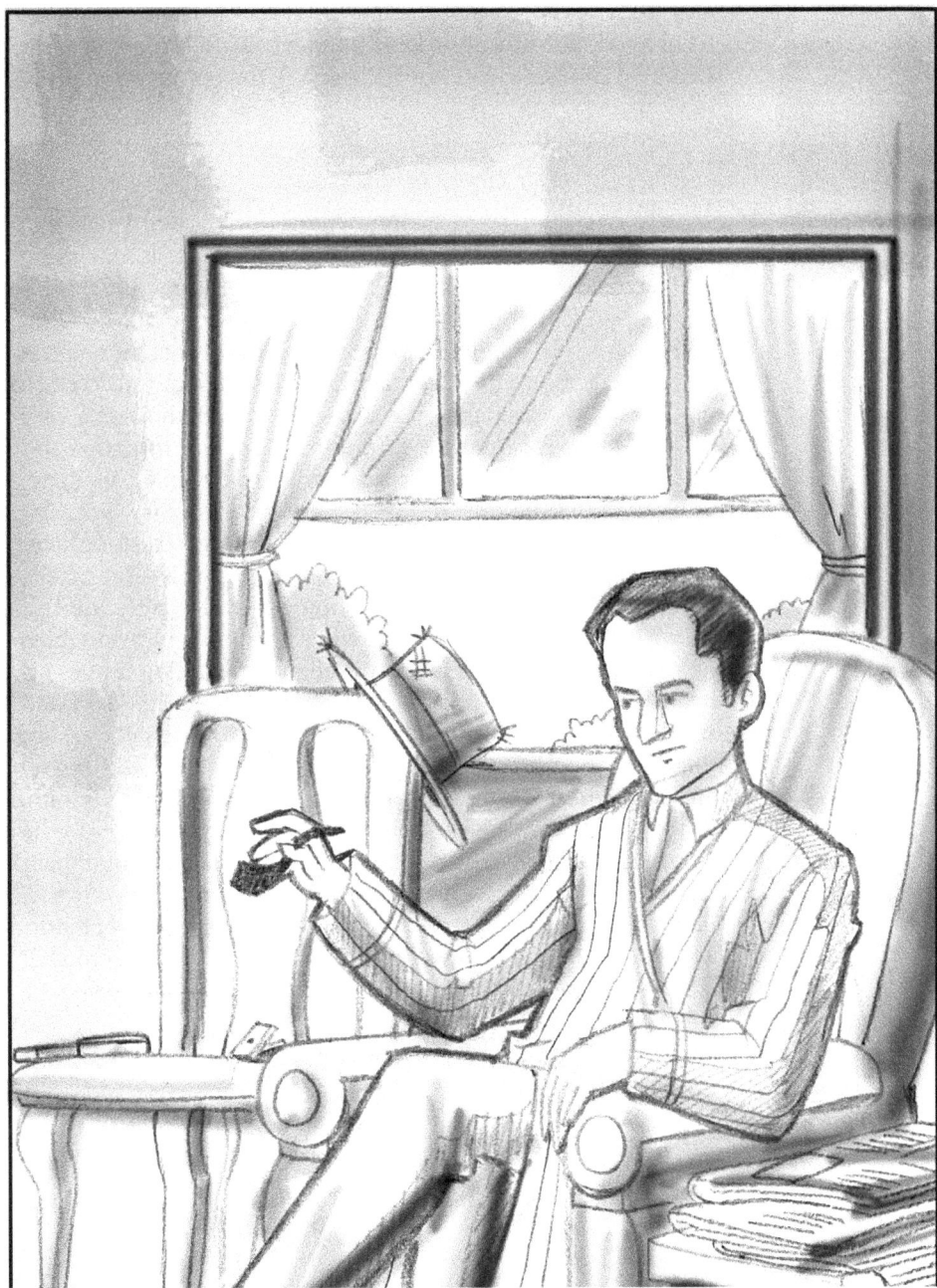

"Precisely. You allude to my attempt to recover the Irene Adler papers, to the singular case of Miss Mary Sutherland, and to the adventure of the man with the twisted lip. Well, I have no doubt that this small matter will fall into the same innocent category. You know Peterson, the commissionaire?"

"Yes."

"It is to him that this trophy belongs."

"It is his hat."

"No, no, he found it. Its owner is unknown. I beg that you will look upon it not as a battered *billycock,* but as an intellectual problem. And, first, as to how it came here. It arrived upon Christmas morning, in company with a good fat goose, which is, I have no doubt, roasting at this moment in front of Peterson's fire. The facts are these: about four o'clock on Christmas morning, Peterson, who, as you know, is a very honest fellow, was returning from some small *jollification* and was making his way homeward down Tottenham Court Road. In front of him he saw, in the gaslight, a tallish man, walking with a slight, stagger, and carrying a white goose slung over his shoulder. As he reached the corner of the Goodge Street, a row broke out between this stranger and a little knot of roughs. One of the latter, knocked off the man's hat, on which he raised his stick to defend himself and, swinging it over his head, smashed the shop window behind him. Peterson had rushed forward to protect the stranger from his assailants; but the man, shocked at having broken the window, and seeing an official-looking person in uniform rushing towards him, dropped his goose, took to his heels, and vanished amid the labyrinth of small streets which lie at the back of Tottenham Court Road. The roughs had also fled at the appearance of Peterson, so that he was left in possession of the field of battle, and also of the spoils of victory in the shape of this battered hat and a most *unimpeachable* Christmas goose."

"Which surely he restored to their owner?"

"My dear fellow, there lies the problem. It is true that 'For Mrs. Henry Baker' was printed upon a small card which was tied to the bird's left leg, and it is also true that the initials 'H. B.' are legible upon the lining of this hat, but as there are some thousands of Bakers, and some hundreds of Henry Bakers in this city of ours, it is not easy to restore lost property to any one of them."

Unimpeachable -
Above suspicion
Billycock – *A kind of a felt-hat*
Jollification –
Merry-making

"What, then, did Peterson do?"

"He brought around both the hat and goose me on the Christmas morning, knowing that even the smallest problems are of interest to me. The goose we retained until this morning, when there were signs that, in spite of the slight frost, it would be well that it should be eaten without unnecessary delay. Its finder has carried it off, therefore, to fulfil the ultimate destiny of a goose, while I continue to retain the hat of the unknown gentleman who lost his Christmas dinner."

"Did he not advertise?"

"No."

"Then, what clue could you have as to his identity?"

"Only as much as we can deduce."

"From his hat?"

"Precisely."

"But you are joking. What can you gather from this old *battered* felt?"

"Here is my lens. You know my methods. What can you gather yourself as to the individuality of the man who has worn this article?"

I took the *tattered* object in my hands and turned it over rather *ruefully*. It was a very ordinary black hat of the usual round shape, hard and much the worse for wear. The lining had been of red silk, but was a good deal discoloured. There was no maker's name; but, as Holmes had remarked, the initials "H. B." were *scrawled* upon one side. It was pierced in the brim for a hat-securer, but the elastic was missing. For the rest, it was cracked, exceedingly dusty, and spotted in several places, although there seemed to have been some attempt to hide the discoloured patches by smearing them with ink.

"I can see nothing," said I, handing it back to my friend.

"On the contrary, Watson, you can see everything. You fail, however, to reason from what you see. You are too timid in drawing your inferences."

"Then, pray tell me what it is that you can infer from this hat?"

He picked it up and gazed at it in the peculiar *introspective* fashion which was characteristic of him. "It is perhaps less suggestive than it might have been," he remarked, "and

Battered - *Badly damaged*
Ruefully - *Causing sorrow or pity*
Inferences - *Conclusions*
Scrawled - *Scribbled*
Tattered – *Torn and old*
Introspective – *Thoughtful*

yet there are a few inferences which are very distinct, and a few others which represent at least a strong balance of probability. That the man was highly intellectual is of course obvious upon the face of it, and also that he was fairly well-to-do within the last three years, although he has now fallen upon evil days. He had *foresight*, but has less now than formerly, pointing to a moral *retrogression*, which, when taken with the decline of his fortunes, seems to indicate some evil influence, probably drink, at work upon him. This may account also for the obvious fact that his wife has ceased to love him."

"My dear Holmes!"

"He has, however, retained some degree of self-respect," he continued, disregarding my *remonstrance*. "He is a man who leads a sedentary life, goes out little, is out of training entirely, is middle-aged, has grizzled hair which he has had cut within the last few days, and which he *anoints* with lime-cream. These are the more patent facts which are to be deduced from his hat. Also, by the way, that it is extremely improbable that he has gas laid on in his house."

"You are certainly joking, Holmes."

"Not in the least. Is it possible that even now, when I give you these results, you are unable to see how they are attained?"

"I have no doubt that I am very stupid, but I must confess that I am unable to follow you. For example, how did you deduce that this man was an intellectual?"

For answer, Holmes clapped the hat upon his head. It came right over the forehead and settled upon the bridge of his nose. "It is a question of cubic capacity," said he; "a man with so large a brain must have something in it."

"The decline of his fortunes, then?"

"This hat is three years old. These flat brims curled at the edge came in then. It is a hat of the very best quality. Look at the band of ribbed silk and the excellent lining. If this man could afford to buy so expensive a hat three years ago, and has had no hat since, then he has assuredly gone down in the world."

"Well, that is clear enough, certainly. But how about the foresight and the moral retrogression?" Sherlock Holmes laughed. "Here is the foresight," said he putting his finger upon the little disc and loop of the hat-securer. "They are never sold upon hats. If this man ordered one, it is a sign of

Foresight - *Care or provision for the future*
Anoints - *To rub or sprinkle on*
Retrogression – *The act of declining or becoming worse*
Remonstrance – *Protest*

a certain amount of foresight, since he went out of his way to take this precaution against the wind. But since we see that he has broken the elastic and has not troubled to replace it, it is obvious that he has less foresight now than formerly, which is a distinct proof of a weakening nature. On the other hand, he has endeavoured to conceal some of these stains upon the felt by *daubing* them with ink, which is a sign that he has not entirely lost his self-respect."

"Your reasoning is certainly *plausible*."

"The further points, that he is middle-aged, that his hair is grizzled, that it has been recently cut, and that he uses limecream, are all to be gathered from a close examination of the lower part of the lining. The lens discloses a large number of hair-ends, clean cut by the scissors of the barber. They all appear to be adhesive, and there is a distinct odour of lime-cream. This dust, you will observe, is not the gritty, gray dust of the street but the fluffy brown dust of the house, showing that it has been hung up indoors most of the time, while the marks of moisture upon the inside are proof positive that the wearer perspired very freely, and could therefore, hardly be in the best of training."

"But his wife – you said that she had ceased to love him."

"This hat has not been brushed for weeks. When I see you, my dear Watson, with a week's accumulation of dust upon your hat, and when your wife allows you to go out in such a state, I shall fear that you also have been unfortunate enough to lose your wife's affection."

"But he might be a bachelor."

"Nay, he was bringing home the goose as a peace-offering to his wife. Remember the card upon the bird's leg."

"You have an answer to everything. But how on earth do you deduce that the gas is not laid on in his house?"

"One tallow stain, or even two, might come by chance; but when I see no less than five, I think that there can be little doubt that the individual must be brought into frequent contact with burning *tallow* – walks upstairs at night probably with his hat in one hand and a guttering candle in the other. Anyhow, he never got tallow-stains from a gas-jet. Are you satisfied?"

"Well, it is very *ingenious*," said I, laughing; "but since, as you said just now, there has been no crime committed, and no

Ingenious - *Showing intelligence*
Plausible - *Well spoken and apparently*
Daubing – *Smearing*
Tallow – *A fatty substance used in making candles*

harm done save the loss of a goose, all this seems to be rather a waste of energy."

Sherlock Holmes had opened his mouth to reply, when the door flew open, and Peterson, the commissionaire, rushed into the apartment with flushed cheeks and the face of a man who is dazed with astonishment.

"The goose, Mr. Holmes! The goose, sir!" he gasped.

"Eh? What of it, then? Has it returned to life and flapped off through the kitchen window?" Holmes twisted himself around upon the sofa to get a fairer view of the man's excited face.

"See here, sir! See what my wife found in its *crop*!" He held out his hand and displayed upon the centre of the palm a brilliantly *scintillating* blue stone, rather smaller than a bean in size, but of such purity and radiance that it twinkled like an electric point in the dark hollow of his hand.

Sherlock Holmes sat up with a whistle. "By Jove, Peterson!" said he, "this is treasure trove indeed. I suppose you know what you have got?"

"A diamond, sir? A precious stone. It cuts into glass as though it were *putty*."

"It's more than a precious stone. It is the precious stone."

"Not the Countess of Morcar's blue carbuncle!" I ejaculated.

"Precisely so. I ought to know its size and shape, seeing that I have read the advertisement about it in *The Times* every day lately. It is absolutely unique, and its value can only be *conjectured*, but the reward offered of 1000 pounds is certainly not within a twentieth part of the market price."

"A thousand pounds! Great Lord of mercy!" The commissionaire plumped down into a chair and stared from one to the other of us.

"That is the reward, and I have reason to know that there are sentimental considerations in the background which would induce the Countess to part with half her fortune if she could but recover the gem."

"It was lost, if I remember aright, at the Hotel Cosmopolitan," I remarked.

"Precisely so, on December 22nd, just five days ago. John Horner, a plumber, was accused of having abstracted it from the lady's jewel-case. The evidence against him was so

Conjectured - *Guessed, Speculated*
Crop – *A part of bird's throat*
Putty – *A substance used for fixing glasses, etc.*

strong that the case has been referred to the Assizes. I have some account of the matter here, I believe." He *rummaged* amid his newspapers, glancing over the dates, until at last he smoothed one out, doubled it over, and read the following paragraph:

"Hotel Cosmopolitan Jewel Robbery. John Horner, 26, plumber, was brought up upon the charge of having upon the 22nd inst., abstracted from the jewel-case of the Countess of Morcar the valuable gem known as the *blue carbuncle*. James Ryder, upper-attendant at the hotel, gave his evidence to the effect that he had shown Horner up to the dressing-room of the Countess of Morcar upon the day of the robbery in order that he might *solder* the second bar of the grate, which was loose. He had remained with Horner some little time, but had finally been called away. On returning, he found that Horner had disappeared, that the bureau had been forced open, and that the small morocco casket in which, as it afterwards transpired, the Countess was accustomed to keep her jewel, was lying empty upon the dressing-table. Ryder instantly gave the alarm, and Horner was arrested the same evening; but the stone could not be found either upon his person or in his rooms. Catherine Cusack, maid to the Countess, *deposed* to having heard Ryder's cry of dismay on discovering the robbery, and to having rushed into the room, where she found matters as described by the last witness. Inspector Bradstreet, B division, gave evidence as to the arrest of Horner, who struggled frantically, and protested his innocence in the strongest terms. Evidence of a previous *conviction* for robbery having been given against the prisoner, the magistrate refused to deal summarily with the offence, but referred it to the Assizes. Horner, who had shown signs of intense emotion during the proceedings, fainted away at the conclusion and was carried out of court.

"Hum! So much for the police-court," said Holmes thoughtfully, tossing aside the paper. "The question for us now to solve is the sequence of events leading from a rifled jewel-case at one end to the crop of a goose in Tottenham Court Road at the other. You see, Watson, our little deductions have suddenly assumed a much more important and less innocent aspect. Here is the stone; the stone came from the goose, and the goose came from Mr. Henry Baker, the gentleman with the bad hat and all the other characteristics with which I have bored you. So now, we must set ourselves

Conviction - *A fixed or firm belief*
Deposed - *To remove from office or position*
Rummaged – *Looked through*
Solder – *Repair, To mend, Patch up*

very seriously to finding this gentleman and ascertaining what part he has played in this little mystery. To do this, we must try the simplest means first, and these lie undoubtedly in an advertisement in all the evening papers. If this fail, I shall have *recourse* to other methods."

"What will you say?"

"Give me a pencil and that slip of paper. Now, then: 'Found at the corner of Goodge Street, a goose and a black felt hat. Mr. Henry Baker can have the same by applying at 6:30 this evening at 221B, Baker Street.' That is clear and concise."

"Very. But will he see it?"

"Well, he is sure to keep an eye on the papers, since, to a poor man, the loss was a heavy one. He was clearly so scared by his mischance in breaking the window and by the approach of Peterson that he thought of nothing but flight, but since then, he must have bitterly regretted the impulse which caused him to drop his bird. Then, again, the introduction of his name will cause him to see it, for everyone who knows him will direct his attention to it. Here you are, Peterson, run down to the advertising agency and have this put in the evening papers."

"In which, sir?"

"Oh, in the Globe, Star, Pall Mall, St. James's, Evening News Standard, Echo, and any others that occur to you."

"Very well, sir. And this stone?"

"Ah, yes, I shall keep the stone. Thank you. And, I say, Peterson, just buy a goose on your way back and leave it here with me, for we must have one to give to this gentleman in place of the one which your family is now *devouring*."

When the commissionaire had gone, Holmes took up the stone and held it against the light. "It's a *bonny* thing," said he. "Just see how it glints and sparkles. Of course, it is a nucleus and focus of crime. Every good stone is. They are the devil's pet baits. In the larger and older jewels, every facet may stand for a bloody deed. This stone is not yet twenty years old. It was found in the banks of the Amoy River in southern China and is remarkable in having every characteristic of the carbuncle, save that it is blue in shade instead of ruby red. In spite of its youth, it has already a *sinister* history. There have been two murders, a vitriol-throwing, a suicide, and several robberies brought about for the sake of this forty-grain weight

Devouring - *To swallow or eat up hungrily*
Recourse – *Route or way*
Bonny – *Attractive*

of crystallized charcoal. Who would think that so pretty a toy would be a *purveyor* to the *gallows* and the prison? I'll lock it up in my strong box now and drop a line to the Countess to say that we have it."

"Do you think that this man Horner is innocent?"

"I cannot tell."

"Well, then, do you imagine that this other one, Henry Baker, had anything to do with the matter?"

"It is, I think, much more likely that Henry Baker is an absolutely innocent man, who had no idea that the bird which he was carrying was of considerably more value than if it were made of solid gold. That, however, I shall determine by a very simple test if we have an answer to our advertisement."

"And you can do nothing until then?"

"Nothing."

"In that case, I shall continue my professional round. But I shall come back in the evening at the hour you have mentioned, for I should like to see the solution of so *tangled* a business."

"Very glad to see you. I dine at seven. There is a woodcock, I believe. By the way, in view of recent occurrences, perhaps, I ought to ask Mrs. Hudson to examine its crop."

I had been delayed at a case, and it was a little after half-past six when I found myself in Baker Street once more. As I approached the house, I saw a tall man in a Scotch bonnet with a coat which was buttoned up to his chin waiting outside in the bright semicircle which was thrown from the fanlight. Just as l arrived, the door was opened, and we were shown up together to Holmes's room.

"Mr. Henry Baker, I believe," said he, rising from his arm-chair and greeting his visitor with the easy air of *geniality* which he could so readily assume. "Pray take this chair by the fire, Mr. Baker. It is a cold night, and I observe that your circulation is more adapted for summer than for winter. Ah, Watson, you have just come at the right time. Is that your hat, Mr. Baker?"

"Yes, sir, that is undoubtedly my hat."

He was a large man with rounded shoulders, a massive head, and a broad, intelligent face, sloping down to a pointed beard of grizzled brown. A touch of red in nose and cheeks, with a slight tremor of his extended hand, recalled Holmes's

Tangled - *Interlaced or complicated*
Bonnet - *A hat usually tied under the chin*
Surmise - *Guess, conjecture*
Purveyor – *Supplier*
Gallows – *A structure where criminals are executed*

surmise as to his habits. His rusty black frock-coat was buttoned right up in front, with the collar turned up, and his **lank** wrists protruded from his sleeves without a sign of cuff or shirt. He spoke in a slow *staccato* fashion, choosing his words with care, and gave the impression generally of a man of learning and letters who had had ill-usage at the hands of fortune.

"We have retained these things for some days," said Holmes, "because we expected to see an advertisement from you giving your address. I am at a loss to know now why you did not advertise."

Our visitor gave a rather shamefaced laugh. "Shillings have not been so plentiful with me as they once were," he remarked. "I had no doubt that the gang of roughs who assaulted me had carried off both my hat and the bird. I did not care to spend more money in a hopeless attempt at recovering them."

"Very naturally. By the way, about the bird, we were compelled to eat it."

"To eat it!" Our visitor half rose from his chair in his excitement.

"Yes, it would have been of no use to anyone had we not done so. But I presume that this other goose upon the sideboard, which is about the same weight and perfectly fresh, will answer your purpose equally well?"

"Oh, certainly, certainly," answered Mr. Baker with a sigh of relief.

"Of course, we still have the feathers, legs, crop, and so on of your own bird, so if you wish –"

The man burst into a hearty laugh. "They might be useful to me as relics of my adventure," said he, "but beyond that I can hardly see what use the disjecta membra of my late acquaintance are going to be to me. No, sir, I think that, with your permission, I will confine my attentions to the excellent bird which I perceive upon the sideboard."

Sherlock Holmes glanced sharply across at me with a slight shrug of his shoulders.

"There is your hat, then, and there your bird," said he. "By the way, would it bore you to tell me where you got the other one from? I am somewhat of a fowl fancier, and I have seldom seen a better grown goose."

"Certainly, sir," said Baker, who had risen and tucked his newly gained property under his arm. "There are a few of

Lank – *Lifeless*
Staccato – *Disjointed*

us who frequent the Alpha Inn, near the Museum – we are to be found in the Museum itself during the day, you understand. This year our good host, Windigate by name, *instituted* a goose club, by which, on consideration of some few pence every week, we were each to receive a bird at Christmas. My pence were duly paid, and the rest is familiar to you. I am much indebted to you, sir, for a Scotch bonnet is fitted neither to my years nor my gravity." With a comical *pomposity* of manner he bowed solemnly to both of us and strode off upon his way.

"So much for Mr. Henry Baker," said Holmes when he had closed the door behind him. "It is quite certain that he knows nothing whatever about the matter. Are you hungry, Watson?"

"Not particularly."

"Then I suggest that we turn our dinner into a supper and follow up this clue while it is still hot."

"By all means."

It was a bitter night, so we drew on our *ulsters* and wrapped *cravats* about our throats. Outside, the stars were shining coldly in a cloudless sky, and the breath of the passers-by blew out into smoke like so many pistol shots. Our footfalls rang out crisply and loudly as we swung through the doctors' quarter, Wimpole Street, Harley Street, and so through Wigmore Street into Oxford Street. In a quarter of an hour, we were in Bloomsbury at the Alpha Inn, which is a small public-house at the corner of one of the streets which runs down into Holborn. Holmes pushed open the door of the private bar and ordered two glasses of beer from the ruddy-faced, white-aproned landlord.

"Your beer should be excellent if it is as good as your geese," said he.

"My geese!" The man seemed surprised.

"Yes. I was speaking only half an hour ago to Mr. Henry Baker, who was a member of your goose club."

"Ah! yes, I see. But you see, sir, them's not our geese."

"Indeed! Whose, then?"

"Well, I got the two dozen from a salesman in Covent Garden."

"Indeed? I know some of them. Which was it?"

"Breckinridge is his name."

Ulsters - *A province in the Northern Republic of Ireland*
Cravats - *Necktie*
Instituted – *Established*
Pomposity – *Arrogance*

"Ah! I don't know him. Well, here's your good health land-lord, and prosperity to your house. Goodnight.

"Now for Mr. Breckinridge," he continued, buttoning up his coat as we came out into the frosty air. "Remember, Watson that though we have so homely a thing as a goose at one end of this chain, we have at the other, a man who will certainly get seven years' penal *servitude* unless we can establish his innocence. It is possible that our inquiry may but confirm his guilt but, in any case, we have a line of investigation which has been missed by the police, and which a singular chance has placed in our hands. Let us follow it out to the bitter end. Faces to the south, then, and quick march!"

We passed across Holborn, down Endell Street, and so through a zigzag of slums to Covent Garden Market. One of the largest stalls bore the name of Breckinridge upon it, and the proprietor a horsy-looking man, with a sharp face and trim side-whiskers was helping a boy to put up the shutters.

"Goodevening. It's a cold night," said Holmes.

The salesman nodded and shot a questioning glance at my companion.

"Sold out of geese, I see," continued Holmes, pointing at the bare slabs of marble.

"Let you have five hundred tomorrow morning."

"That's no good."

"Well, there are some on the stall with the gas-flare."

"Ah, but I was recommended to you."

"Who by?"

"The landlord of the Alpha."

"Oh, yes; I sent him a couple of dozen."

"Fine birds they were, too. Now where did you get them from?"

To my surprise the question provoked a burst of anger from the salesman.

"Now, then, mister," said he, with his head *cocked* and his arms *akimbo*, "what are you driving at? Let's have it straight, now."

Cocked – *Raised (an eye or an ear) at someone*
Akimbo – *With hands on the hips and elbows outward*

"It is straight enough. I should like to know who sold you the geese which you supplied to the Alpha."

"Well then, I shan't tell you. So now!"

Greatest Adventure Stories of Sherlock Holmes - 2

"Oh, it is a matter of no importance; but I don't know why you should be so warm over such a trifle."

"Warm! You'd be as warm, maybe, if you were as **pestered** as I am. When I pay good money for a good article there should be an end of the business; but it's 'Where are the geese?' and 'Who did you sell the geese to?' and 'What will you take for the geese?' One would think they were the only geese in the world, to hear the fuss that is made over them."

"Well, I have no connection with any other people who have been making inquiries," said Holmes carelessly. "If you won't tell us the bet is off, that is all. But I'm always ready to back my opinion on a matter of fowls, and I have a fiver on it that the bird I ate is country bred."

"Well, then, you've lost your fiver, for it's town bred," snapped the salesman.

"It's nothing of the kind."

"I say it is."

"I don't believe it."

"D'you think you know more about fowls than I, who have handled them ever since I was a **nipper**? I tell you, all those birds that went to the Alpha were town bred."

"You'll never persuade me to believe that."

"Will you bet, then?"

"It's merely taking your money, for I know that I am right. But I'll have a sovereign on with you, just to teach you not to be obstinate."

The salesman chuckled grimly. "Bring me the books, Bill," said he.

The small boy brought around a small thin volume and a great greasy-backed one, laying them out together beneath the hanging lamp.

"Now then, Mr. Cocksure," said the salesman, "I thought that I was out of geese, but before I finish you'll find that there is still one left in my shop. You see this little book?"

"Well?"

"That's the list of the folk from whom I buy. D'you see? Well, then, here on this page are the country folk, and the numbers after their names are where their accounts are in the big ledger. Now, then! You see this other page in red ink? Well, that is a list of my town suppliers. Now, look at that third name. Just read it out to me."

Ledger - *An account book of final entry*
Fiver - *A five - dollar bill*
Pestered – *Bothered*
Nipper – *A small child*

"Mrs. Oakshott, 117, Brixton Road – 249," read Holmes.

"Quite so. Now turn that up in the ledger."

Holmes turned to the page indicated. "Here you are, 'Mrs. Oakshott, 117, Brixton Road, egg and poultry supplier.'"

"Now, then, what's the last entry?"

"'December 22nd. Twenty-four geese at 7s. 6d.'"

"Quite so. There you are. And underneath?"

"'Sold to Mr. Windigate of the Alpha, at 12s.'"

"What have you to say now?"

Sherlock Holmes looked deeply **chagrined**. He drew a sovereign from his pocket and threw it down upon the slab, turning away with the air of a man whose disgust is too deep for words. A few yards off he stopped under a lamp-post and laughed in the hearty, noiseless fashion which was peculiar to him.

"When you see a man with whiskers of that cut and the 'Pink 'un' protruding out of his pocket, you can always draw him by a bet," said he. "I daresay that if I had put 100 pounds down in front of him, that man would not have given me such complete information as was drawn from him by the idea that he was doing me on a wager. Well, Watson, we are, I fancy, nearing the end of our quest, and the only point which remains to be determined is whether we should go on to this Mrs. Oakshott tonight, or whether we should reserve it for tomorrow. It is clear from what that **surly** fellow said that there are others besides ourselves who are anxious about the matter, and I should –"

His remarks were suddenly cut short by a loud hubbub which broke out from the stall which we had just left. Turning around, we saw a little rat-faced fellow standing in the centre of the circle of yellow light which was thrown by the swinging lamp, while Breckinridge, the salesman, framed in the door of his stall, was shaking his fists fiercely at the **cringing** figure.

"I've had enough of you and your geese," he shouted. "I wish you were all at the devil together. If you come **pestering** me any more with your silly talk, I'll set the dog at you. You bring Mrs. Oakshott here and I'll answer her, but what have you to do with it? Did I buy the geese off you?"

"No; but one of them was mine all the same," whined the little man.

"Well, then, ask Mrs. Oakshott for it."

Pestering - *To bother persistently*
Cringing - *Shrinking*
Chagrined – *Annoyed*
Surly – *Rude, Bad tempered*

"She told me to ask you."

"Well, you can ask the King of Proosia, for all I care. I've had enough of it. Get out of this!" He rushed fiercely forward, and the inquirer *flitted away* into the darkness.

"Ha! this may save us a visit to Brixton Road," whispered Holmes. "Come with me, and we will see what is to be made of this fellow." Striding through the scattered knots of people who lounged around the flaring stalls, my companion speedily overtook the little man and touched him upon the shoulder. He sprang around, and I could see in the gas-light that every vestige of colour had been driven from his face.

"Who are you, then? What do you want?" he asked in a *quavering* voice.

"You will excuse me," said Holmes *blandly*, "but I could not help overhearing the questions which you put to the salesman just now. I think that I could be of assistance to you."

"You? Who are you? How could you know anything of the matter?"

"My name is Sherlock Holmes. It is my business to know what other people don't know."

"But you can know nothing of this?'"

"Excuse me, I know everything of it. You are endeavouring to trace some geese which were sold by Mrs. Oakshott, of Brixton Road, to a salesman named Breckinridge, by him in turn to Mr. Windigate, of the Alpha, and by him to his club, of which Mr. Henry Baker is a member."

"Oh, sir, you are the very man whom I have longed to meet," cried the little fellow with outstretched hands and quivering fingers. "I can hardly explain to you how interested I am in this matter."

Sherlock Holmes hailed a four-wheeler which was passing. "In that case we had better discuss it in a cosy room rather than in this wind-swept market-place," said he. "But pray tell me, before we go farther, who it is that I have the pleasure of assisting."

The man hesitated for an instant. "My name is John Robinson," he answered with a sidelong glance.

"No, no; the real name," said Holmes sweetly. "It is always awkward doing business with an *alias*."

A flush sprang to the white cheeks of the stranger. "Well then," said he, "my real name is James Ryder."

Blandly - *Pleasantly*
Quavering - *Trembling*
Flitted away – *Fade/ Go away*
Alias – *Assumed name*

"Precisely so. Head attendant at the Hotel Cosmopolitan. Pray step into the cab, and I shall soon be able to tell you everything which you would wish to know."

The little man stood glancing from one to the other of us with half-frightened, half-hopeful eyes, as one who is not sure whether he is on the verge of a *windfall* or of a *catastrophe*. Then he stepped into the cab, and in half an hour we were back in the sitting room at Baker Street. Nothing had been said during our drive, but the high, thin breathing of our new companion, and the claspings and unclaspings of his hands, spoke of the nervous tension within him.

"Here we are!" said Holmes cheerily as we filed into the room. "The fire looks very seasonable in this weather. You look cold, Mr. Ryder. Pray take the basket-chair. I will just put on my slippers before we settle this little matter of yours. Now, then! You want to know what became of those geese?"

"Yes, sir."

"Or rather, I fancy, of that goose. It was one bird, I imagine in which you were interested – white, with a black bar across the tail."

Ryder *quivered* with emotion. "Oh, sir," he cried, "can you tell me where it went to?"

"It came here."

"Here?"

"Yes, and a most remarkable bird it proved. I don't wonder that you should take an interest in it. It laid an egg after it was dead – the bonniest, brightest little blue egg that ever was seen. I have it here in my museum."

Our visitor *staggered* to his feet and clutched the mantelpiece with his right hand. Holmes unlocked his strong-box and held up the blue carbuncle, which shone out like a star, with a cold brilliant, many-pointed radiance. Ryder stood glaring with a drawn face, uncertain whether to claim or to disown it.

"The game's up, Ryder," said Holmes quietly. "Hold up, man, or you'll be into the fire! Give him an arm back into his chair, Watson. He's not got blood enough to go in for *felony* with *impunity*. Give him a dash of brandy. So! Now he looks a little more human. What a **shrimp** it is, to be sure!"

For a moment, he had staggered and nearly fallen, but the brandy brought a tinge of colour into his cheeks, and he sat staring with frightened eyes at his accuser.

Felony - *An offence*
Staggered - *To walk, move, or stand unsteadily*
Impunity - *Exemption from punishment*
Windfall – *An unexpected gain, Good fortune*
Shrimp – *A marine crustacean*

"I have almost every link in my hands, and all the proofs which I could possibly need, so there is little which you need to tell me. Still, that little may as well be cleared up to make the case complete. You had heard, Ryder, of this blue stone of the Countess of Morcar's?"

"It was Catherine Cusack who told me of it," said he in a crackling voice.

"I see – her ladyship's waiting-maid. Well, the temptation of sudden wealth so easily acquired was too much for you, as it has been for better men before you; but you were not very *scrupulous* in the means you used. It seems to me, Ryder, that there is the making of a very pretty villain in you. You knew that this man Horner, the plumber, had been concerned in some such matter before, and that suspicion would rest the more readily upon him. What did you do, then? You made some small job in my lady's room – you and your confederate Cusack – and you managed that he should be the man sent for. Then, when he had left, you rifled the jewel-case, raised the alarm, and had this unfortunate man arrested. You then –"

Ryder threw himself down suddenly upon the rug and clutched at my companion's knees. "For God's sake, have mercy!" he shrieked. "Think of my father! of my mother! It would break their hearts. I never went wrong before! I never will again. I swear it. I'll swear it on a Bible. Oh, don't bring it into court! For Christ's sake, don't!"

"Get back into your chair!" said Holmes sternly. "It is very well to cringe and crawl now, but you thought little enough of this poor Horner in the dock for a crime of which he knew nothing."

"I will fly, Mr. Holmes. I will leave the country, sir. Then the charge against him will break down."

"Hum! We will talk about that. And now let us hear a true account of the next act. How came the stone into the goose, and how came the goose into the open market? Tell us the truth, for there lies your only hope of safety."

Ryder passed his tongue over his *parched* lips. "I will tell you it just as it happened, sir," said he. "When Horner had been arrested, it seemed to me that it would be best for me to get away with the stone at once, for I did not know at what moment the police might not take it into their heads to search

Sternly - *Strictly*
Scrupulous –
Conscientious
Parched – *Dry*

me and my room. There was no place about the hotel where it would be safe. I went out, as if on some commission, and I made for my sister's house. She had married a man named Oakshott, and lived in Brixton Road, where she fattened fowls for the market. All the way there every man I met seemed to me to be a policeman or a detective; and, for all that it was a cold night, the sweat was pouring down my face before I came to the Brixton Road. My sister asked me what was the matter, and why I was so pale; but I told her that I had been upset by the jewel robbery at the hotel. Then I went into the backyard and smoked a pipe and wondered what it would be best to do.

"I had a friend once called Maudsley, who went to the bad, and has just been serving his time in Pentonville. One day he had met me, and fell into talk about the ways of thieves, and how they could get rid of what they stole. I knew that he would be true to me, for I knew one or two things about him; so I made up my mind to go right on to Kilburn, where he lived, and take him into my confidence. He would show me how to turn the stone into money. But how to get to him in safety? I thought of the agonies I had gone through in coming from the hotel. I might at any moment be seized and searched, and there would be the stone in my waistcoat pocket. I was leaning against the wall at the time and looking at the geese which were **waddling** about around my feet, and suddenly an idea came into my head which showed me how I could beat the best detective that ever lived.

"My sister had told me some weeks before that I might have the pick of her geese for a Christmas present, and I knew that she was always as good as her word. I would take my goose now, and in it I would carry my stone to Kilburn. There was a little shed in the yard, and behind this I drove one of the birds – a fine big one, white, with a barred tail. I caught it, and prying its bill open, I thrust the stone down its throat as far as my finger could reach. The bird gave a gulp, and I felt the stone pass along its **gullet** and down into its crop. But the creature flapped and struggled, and out came my sister to know what was the matter. As I turned to speak to her, the brute broke loose and fluttered off among the others.

"'Whatever were you doing with that bird, Jem?' says she.

"'Well,' said I, 'you said you'd give me one for Christmas, and I was feeling which was the fattest.'

Waddling – *Swaying*
Gullet – *Throat*

"'Oh,' says she, 'we've set yours aside for you – Jem's bird, we call it. It's the big white one over yonder. There's twenty-six of them, which makes one for you, and one for us, and two dozen for the market.'

"'Thank you, Maggie,' said I; 'but if it is all the same to you, I'd rather have that one I was handling just now.'

"'The other is a good three pound heavier,' said she, 'and we fattened it expressly for you.'

"'Never mind. I'll have the other, and I'll take it now,' said I.

"'Oh, just as you like,' said she, a little *huffed*. 'Which is it you want, then?'

"'That white one with the barred tail, right in the middle of the flock.'

"'Oh, very well. Kill it and take it with you.'

"Well, I did what she said, Mr. Holmes, and I carried the bird all the way to Kilburn. I told my *pal* what I had done, for he was a man that it was easy to tell a thing like that to. He laughed until he choked, and we got a knife and opened the goose. My heart turned to water, for there was no sign of the stone, and I knew that some terrible mistake had occurred. I left the bird rushed back to my sister's, and hurried into the backyard. There was not a bird to be seen there.

"'Where are they all, Maggie?' I cried.

"'Gone to the dealer's, Jem.'

"'Which dealer's?'

"'Breckinridge, of Covent Garden.'

"'But was there another with a barred tail?' I asked, 'The same as the one I chose?'

"'Yes, Jem; there were two barred-tailed ones, and I could never tell them apart.'

"Well, then, of course I saw it all, and I ran off as hard as my feet would carry me to this man Breckinridge; but he had sold the lot at once, and not one word would he tell me as to where they had gone. You heard him yourselves tonight. Well, he has always answered me like that. My sister thinks that I am going mad. Sometimes, I think that I am myself. And now – and now I am myself a branded thief, without ever having touched the wealth for which I sold my character. God help me! God help me!" He burst into *convulsive* sobbing, with his face buried in his hands.

Pal - *Friend*
Huffed – *Gasped*
Convulsive – *Bursting*

There was a long silence, broken only by his heavy breathing and by the measured tapping of Sherlock Holmes's fingertips upon the edge of the table. Then my friend rose and threw open the door.

"Get out!" said he.

"What, sir! Oh, Heaven bless you!"

"No more words. Get out!"

And no more words were needed. There was a rush, a clatter upon the stairs, the bang of a door, and the crisp rattle of running *footfalls* from the street.

"After all, Watson," said Holmes, reaching up his hand for his clay pipe, "I am not retained by the police to supply their *deficiencies*. If Horner were in danger, it would be another thing; but this fellow will not appear against him, and the case must collapse. I suppose that I am *commuting* a *felony*. but it is just possible that I am saving a soul. This fellow will not go wrong again; he is too terribly frightened. Send him to jail now, and you make him a jail-bird for life. Besides, it is the season of forgiveness. Chance has put in our way a most singular and whimsical problem, and its solution is its own reward. If you will have the goodness to touch the bell, Doctor, we will begin another investigation, in which, also a bird will be the chief feature."

Footfalls – *Sound of footsteps*
Commuting – *Travelling*
Felony - *A serious crime*
Deficiencies - *Scarcity, Shortage*

Food For Thought

Why did Holmes order the guilty, James Ryder to get out of the place? What would have happened if Holmes would not have set Ryder free?

An Understanding

Q. 1. How did Holmes draw inferences about the individuality of the man who wore the tattered, very ordinary looking black hat, while Watson failed to do so?

Ans. _____

_____

_____

_____

_____

Q. 2. "It's more than a precious stone. It is the precious stone." Who said these words to whom? What was the name of the precious stone and whom did it belong to?

Ans. _____

_____

_____

_____

_____

Q. 3. Where did the commissionaire Peterson find the sparkling 'Blue Carbuncle'? When and from where was it stolen? What was the reward offered on it?

Ans. _____

_____

_____

_____

_____

Q. 4. How did Holmes catch the thief, who stole the precious 'Blue Carbuncle'? What was his actual name? How did the thief manage to get his hands on the invaluable gem?

Ans. _____

_____

_____

_____

_____

The Adventure of the Beryl Coronet

~ Arthur Conan Doyle

"Holmes," said I as I stood one morning in our bow-window looking down the street, "here is a mad man coming along. It seems rather sad that his relatives should allow him to come out alone."

My friend rose lazily from his armchair and stood with his hands in the pockets of his dressing-gown, looking over my shoulder. It was a bright, crisp February morning, and the snow of the day before still lay deep upon the ground, **shimmering** brightly in the wintry sun. Down the centre of Baker Street, it had been ploughed into a brown crumbly band by the traffic, but at either side and on the heaped-up edges of the footpaths, it still lay as white as when it fell. The grey pavement had been cleaned and scraped, but was still dangerously slippery, so that there were fewer passengers than usual. Indeed, from the direction of the Metropolitan Station, no one was coming save the single gentleman whose eccentric conduct had drawn my attention.

He was a man of about fifty, tall, **portly**, and imposing, with a massive, strongly marked face and a commanding figure. He was dressed in a **sombre**, yet rich style, in black frock-coat, shining hat, neat brown **gaiters**, and well-cut pearl-grey trousers. Yet his actions were in absurd contrast to the dignity of his dress and features, for he was running hard, with occasional little springs, such as a weary man gives who is little accustomed to set any tax upon his legs. As he ran he jerked his hands up and down, **waggled** his head, and **writhed** his face into the most extraordinary **contortions**.

"What on earth can be the matter with him?" I asked. "He is looking up at the numbers of the houses."

"I believe that he is coming here," said Holmes, rubbing his hands.

"Here?"

"Yes; I rather think he is coming to consult me professionally. I think that I recognise the symptoms. Ha! did I not tell you?" As he spoke, the man, puffing and blowing, rushed at our door

Contortions - *Whirling around*
Writhed - *To twist the body*
Waggled - *To wobble or shake*
Gaiters - *Overshoes with fabric tops*
Shimmering - *Shining with faint or dim light*
Portly – *Well-built*
Sombe – *Serious*

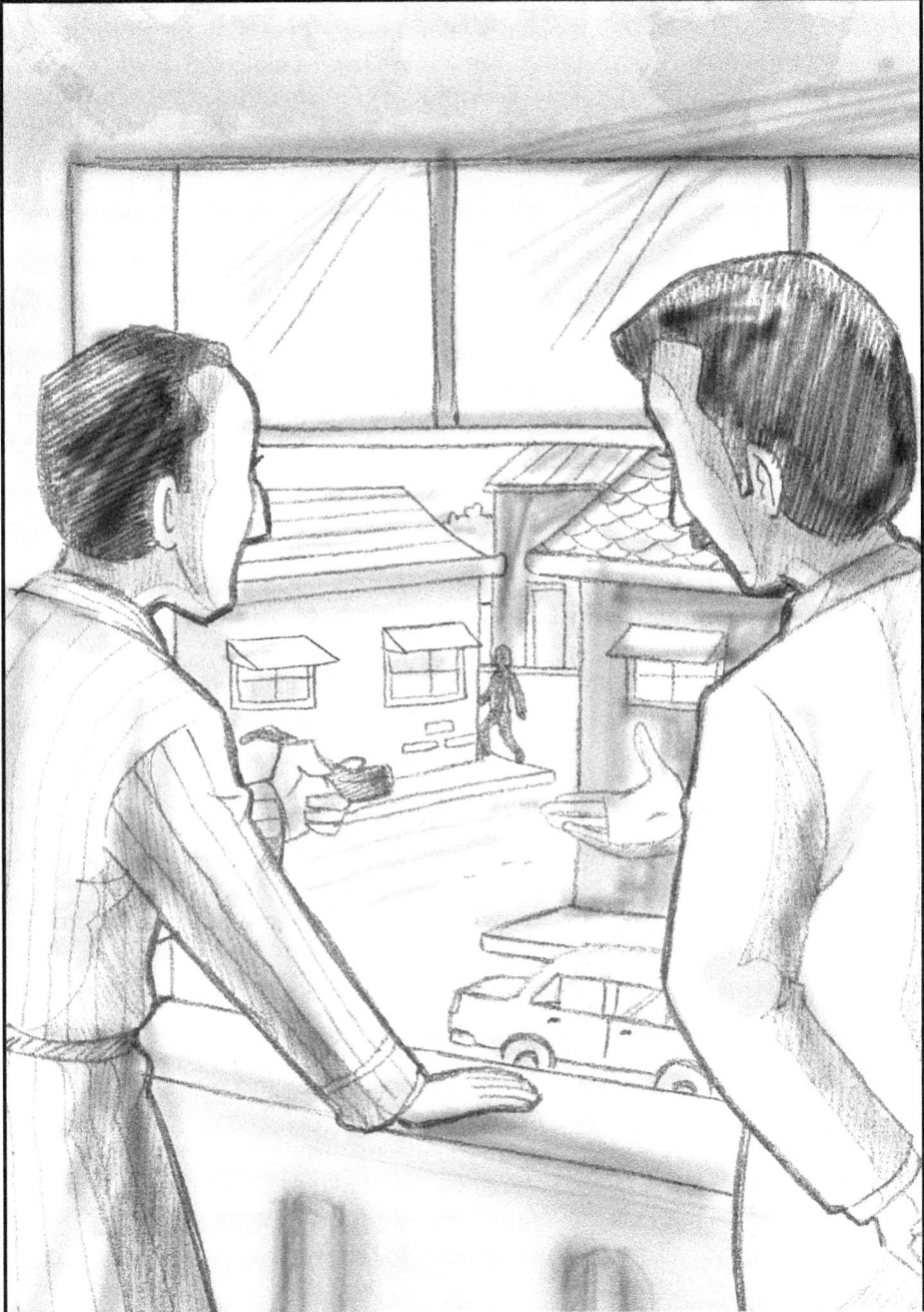

and pulled at our bell until the whole house resounded with the clanging.

A few moments later, he was in our room, still puffing, still *gesticulating*, but with so fixed a look of grief and despair in his eyes that our smiles were turned in an instant to horror and pity. For a while, he could not get his words out, but swayed his body and plucked at his hair like one who has been driven to the extreme limits of his reason. Then, suddenly springing to his feet, he beat his head against the wall with such force that we both rushed upon him and tore him away to the centre of the room. Sherlock Holmes pushed him down into the easy-chair and, sitting beside him, patted his hand and chatted with him in the easy, soothing tones which he knew so well how to employ.

"You have come to me to tell your story, have you not?" said he. "You are fatigued with your haste. Pray wait until you have recovered yourself, and then I shall be most happy to look into any little problem which you may submit to me."

The man sat for a minute or more with a *heaving* chest, fighting against his emotion. Then he passed his handkerchief over his brow, set his lips tight, and turned his face towards us.

"No doubt you think me mad?" said he.

"I see that you have had some great trouble," responded Holmes.

"God knows I have! – a trouble which is enough to unseat my reason, so sudden and so terrible it is. Public disgrace, I might have faced, although I am a man whose character has never yet borne a stain. Private *affliction* also is the lot of every man; but the two coming together, and in so frightful a form, have been enough to shake my very soul. Besides, it is not I alone. The very noblest in the land may suffer unless some way be found out of this horrible affair."

"Pray compose yourself, sir," said Holmes, "and let me have a clear account of who you are and what it is that has *befallen* you."

"My name," answered our visitor, "is probably familiar to your ears. I am Alexander Holder, of the banking firm of Holder & Stevenson, of Threadneedle Street."

The name was indeed well known to us as belonging to the senior partner in the second largest private banking concern

Heaving - *To utter painfully*
Befallen - *Happen by fate or chance*
Gesticulating – *Signalling*
Affliction – *Suffering*

in the City of London. What could have happened, then, to bring one of the foremost citizens of London to this most pitiable pass? We waited, all curiosity, until with another effort, he braced himself to tell his story.

"I feel that time is of value," said he; "that is why I *hastened* here when the police inspector suggested that I should secure your cooperation. I came to Baker Street by the Underground and hurried from there on foot, for the cabs go slowly through this snow. That is why I was so out of breath, for I am a man who takes very little exercise. I feel better now, and I will put the facts before you as shortly and yet as clearly as I can.

"It is, of course, well known to you that in a successful banking business as much depends upon our being able to find *remunerative* investments for our funds as upon our increasing our connection and the number of our depositors. One of our most *lucrative* means of laying out money is in the shape of loans, where the security is *unimpeachable*. We have done a good deal in this direction during the last few years, and there are many noble families to whom we have advanced large sums upon the security of their pictures, libraries, or plate.

"Yesterday morning, I was seated in my office at the bank when a card was brought in to me by one of the clerks. I started when I saw the name, for it was that of none other than – well, perhaps even to you I had better say no more than that it was a name which is a household word all over the earth – one of the highest, noblest, most exalted names in England. I was overwhelmed by the honour and attempted, when he entered, to say so, but he plunged at once into business with the air of a man who wishes to hurry quickly through a disagreeable task.

"'Mr. Holder,' said he, 'I have been informed that you are in the habit of advancing money.'

"'The firm does so when the security is good.' I answered.

"'It is absolutely essential to me,' said he, 'that I should have 50,000 pounds at once. I could, of course, borrow so trifling a sum ten times over from my friends, but I much prefer to make it a matter of business and to carry out that business myself. In my position, you can readily understand that it is unwise to place one's self under obligations.'

"'For how long, may I ask, do you want this sum?' I asked.

"'Next Monday, I have a large sum due to me, and I shall then most certainly repay what you advance, with whatever

Lucrative - *Profitable*
Hastened - *Hurried*
Remunerative –
That pays money
Unimpeachable –
Flawless

interest you think it right to charge. But it is very essential to me that the money should be paid at once.'

"'I should be happy to advance it without further *parley* from my own private purse,' said I, 'were it not that the strain would be rather more than it could bear. If, on the other hand, I am to do it in the name of the firm, then in justice to my partner, I must insist that, even in your case, every businesslike precaution should be taken.'

"'I should much prefer to have it so,' said he, raising up a square, black morocco case which he had laid beside his chair. 'You have doubtless heard of the Beryl Coronet?'

"'One of the most precious public possessions of the empire,' said I.

"'Precisely.' He opened the case, and there, *imbedded* in soft, flesh-coloured velvet, lay the magnificent piece of jewellery which he had named. 'There are thirty-nine enormous beryls,' said he, 'and the price of the gold chasing is incalculable. The lowest estimate would put the worth of the coronet at double the sum which I have asked. I am prepared to leave it with you as my security.'

"I took the precious case into my hands and looked in some perplexity from it to my illustrious client.

"'You doubt its value?' he asked.

"'Not at all. I only doubt –'

"'The *propriety* of my leaving it. You may set your mind at rest about that. I should not dream of doing so were it not absolutely certain that I should be able in four days to reclaim it. It is a pure matter of form. Is the security sufficient?'

"'Ample.'

"'You understand, Mr. Holder, that I am giving you a strong proof of the confidence which I have in you, founded upon all that I have heard of you. I rely upon you not only to be discreet and to refrain from all gossip upon the matter but, above all, to preserve this coronet with every possible precaution because I need not say that a great public scandal would be caused if any harm were to befall it. Any injury to it would be almost as serious as its complete loss, for there are no beryls in the world to match these, and it would be impossible to replace them. I leave it with you, however, with every confidence, and I shall call for it in person on Monday morning.'

Refrain - *Abstain*
Discreet - *Modest and judicious*
Propriety - *Rightness or justness*
Parley – *Discussion*
Imbedded – *Fixed into something*

"Seeing that my client was anxious to leave, I said no more but, calling for my cashier, I ordered him to pay over fifty 1000 pound notes. When I was alone once more, however, with the precious case lying upon the table in front of me, I could not but think with some *misgivings* of the immense responsibility which it *entailed* upon me. There could be no doubt that, as it was a national possession, a horrible scandal would ensue if any misfortune should occur to it. I already regretted having ever consented to take charge of it. However, it was too late to alter the matter now, so I locked it up in my private safe and turned once more to my work.

"When evening came, I felt that it would be an *imprudence* to leave so precious a thing in the office behind me. Bankers' safes had been forced before now, and why should not mine be? If so, how terrible would be the position in which I should find myself! I determined, therefore, that for the next few days, I would always carry the case backward and forward with me, so that it might never be really out of my reach. With this intention, I called a cab and drove out to my house at Streatham, carrying the jewel with me. I did not breathe freely until I had taken it upstairs and locked it in the bureau of my dressing-room.

"And now a word as to my household, Mr. Holmes, for I wish you to thoroughly understand the situation. My groom and my page sleep out of the house, and may be set aside altogether. I have three maidservants who have been with me a number of years and whose absolute reliability is quite above suspicion. Another, Lucy Parr, the second waiting-maid, has only been in my service a few months. She came with an excellent character, however, and has always given me satisfaction. She is a very pretty girl and has attracted admirers who have occasionally hung about the place. That is the only drawback which we have found to her, but we believe her to be a thoroughly good girl in every way.

"So much for the servants. My family itself is so small that it will not take me long to describe it. I am a widower and have an only son, Arthur. He has been a disappointment to me, Mr. Holmes – a grievous disappointment. I have no doubt that I am myself to blame. People tell me that I have spoiled him. Very likely I have. When my dear wife died, I felt that he was all I had to love. I could not bear to see the smile fade even for a moment from his face. I have never denied him a wish.

Entailed - *Imposed*
Misgiving – *Suspicion*
Imprudence – *Innocence*

Perhaps, it would have been better for both of us had I been sterner, but I meant it for the best.

"It was naturally my intention that he should succeed me in my business, but he was not of a business turn. He was wild, *wayward*, and, to speak the truth, I could not trust him in the handling of large sums of money. When he was young he became a member of an aristocratic club, and there, having charming manners, he was soon the intimate of a number of men with long purses and expensive habits. He learned to play heavily at cards and to *squander* money on the *turf*, until he had again and again to come to me and implore me to give him an advance upon his allowance, that he might settle his debts of honour. He tried more than once to break away from the dangerous company which he was keeping, but each time the influence of his friend, Sir George Burnwell, was enough to draw him back again.

"And, indeed, I could not wonder that such a man as Sir George Burnwell should gain an influence over him, for he has frequently brought him to my house, and I have found myself that I could hardly resist the fascination of his manner. He is older than Arthur, a man of the world to his fingertips, one who had been everywhere, seen everything, a brilliant talker, and a man of great personal beauty. Yet when I think of him in cold blood, far away from the glamour of his presence, I am convinced from his cynical speech and the look which I have caught in his eyes that he is one who should be deeply distrusted. So I think, and so, too, thinks my little Mary, who has a woman's quick insight into character.

"And now there is only she to be described. She is my niece; but when my brother died five years ago and left her alone in the world I adopted her, and have looked upon her ever since as my daughter. She is a sunbeam in my house – sweet, loving, beautiful, a wonderful manager and housekeeper, yet as tender and quiet and gentle as a woman could be. She is my right hand. I do not know what I could do without her. In only one matter has she ever gone against my wishes. Twice my boy has asked her to marry him, for he loves her devotedly, but each time, she has refused him. I think that if anyone could have drawn him into the right path, it would have been she, and that his marriage might have changed his whole life; but now, alas! it is too late – forever too late!

Wayward – *Naughty*
Squander – *Waste*

"Now, Mr. Holmes, you know the people who live under my roof, and I shall continue with my miserable story.

"When we were taking coffee in the drawing room that night after dinner, I told Arthur and Mary my experience, and of the precious treasure which we had under our roof, **suppressing** only the name of my client. Lucy Parr, who had brought in the coffee, had, I am sure, left the room; but I cannot swear that the door was closed. Mary and Arthur were much interested and wished to see the famous coronet, but I thought it better not to disturb it.

"'Where have you put it?' asked Arthur.

"'In my own bureau.'

"'Well, I hope to goodness the house won't be burgled during the night.' said he.

"'It is locked up,' I answered.

"'Oh, any old key will fit that bureau. When I was a youngster, I have opened it myself with the key of the box-room cupboard.'

"He often had a wild way of talking, so that I thought little of what he said. He followed me to my room, however, that night with a very grave face.

"'Look here, dad,' said he with his eyes cast down, 'can you let me have 200 pounds?'

"'No, I cannot!' I answered sharply. 'I have been far too generous with you in money matters.'

"'You have been very kind,' said he, 'but I must have this money, or else I can never show my face inside the club again.'

"'And a very good thing, too!' I cried.

"'Yes, but you would not have me leave it a dishonoured man,' said he. 'I could not bear the disgrace. I must raise the money in some way, and if you will not let me have it, then I must try other means.'

"I was very angry, for this was the third demand during the month. 'You shall not have a *farthing* from me,' I cried, on which he bowed and left the room without another word.

"When he was gone, I unlocked my bureau, made sure that my treasure was safe, and locked it again. Then I started to go around the house to see that all was secure – a duty which I usually leave to Mary but which I thought it well to perform myself that night. As I came down the stairs, I saw Mary

Suppressing –
Putting an end to something by force
Farthing – *A British coin (old currency)*

herself at the side window of the hall, which she closed and fastened as I approached.

"'Tell me, dad,' said she, looking, I thought, a little disturbed, 'did you give Lucy, the maid, leave to go out tonight?'

"'Certainly not.'

"'She came in just now by the back door. I have no doubt that she has only been to the side gate to see someone, but I think that it is hardly safe and should be stopped.'

"'You must speak to her in the morning, or I will if you prefer it. Are you sure that everything is *fastened*?'

"'Quite sure, dad.'

"'Then, good night.' I kissed her and went up to my bedroom again, where I was soon asleep.

"I am endeavouring to tell you everything, Mr. Holmes, which may have any bearing upon the case, but I beg that you will question me upon any point which I do not make clear."

"On the contrary, your statement is singularly lucid."

"I come to a part of my story now in which I should wish to be particularly so. I am not a very heavy sleeper, and the anxiety in my mind tended, no doubt, to make me even less so than usual. About two in the morning, then, I was awakened by some sound in the house. It had ceased *ere* I was wide awake, but it had left an impression behind it as though a window had gently closed somewhere. I lay listening with all my ears. Suddenly, to my horror, there was a distinct sound of footsteps moving softly in the next room. I slipped out of bed, all *palpitating* with fear, and peeped round the corner of my dressing-room door.

"'Arthur!' I screamed, 'you villain! you thief! How dare you touch that coronet?'

"The gas was half up, as I had left it, and my unhappy boy, dressed only in his shirt and trousers, was standing beside the light, holding the coronet in his hands. He appeared to be *wrenching* at it, or bending it with all his strength. At my cry he dropped it from his grasp and turned as pale as death. I snatched it up and examined it. One of the gold corners, with three of the beryls in it, was missing.

"'You blackguard!' I shouted, beside myself with rage. 'You have destroyed it! You have *dishonored* me forever! Where are the jewels which you have stolen?'

"'Stolen!' he cried.

Fastened – *Fixed*
Ere – *Before*

"'Yes, thief!' I roared, shaking him by the shoulder.

"'There are none missing. There cannot be any missing,' said he.

"'There are three missing. And you know where they are. Must I call you a liar as well as a thief? Did I not see you trying to tear off another piece?'

"'You have called me names enough,' said he, 'I will not stand it any longer. I shall not say another word about this business, since you have chosen to insult me. I will leave your house in the morning and make my own way in the world.'

"'You shall leave it in the hands of the police!' I cried half-mad with grief and rage. 'I shall have this matter *probed* to the bottom.'

"'You shall learn nothing from me,' said he with a passion such as I should not have thought was in his nature. 'If you choose to call the police, let the police find what they can.'

"By this time, the whole house was *astir*, for I had raised my voice in my anger. Mary was the first to rush into my room, and, at the sight of the coronet and of Arthur's face, she read the whole story and, with a scream, fell down senseless on the ground. I sent the housemaid for the police and put the investigation into their hands at once. When the inspector and a constable entered the house, Arthur, who had stood *sullenly* with his arms folded, asked me whether it was my intention to charge him with theft. I answered that it had ceased to be a private matter, but had become a public one, since the ruined coronet was national property. I was determined that the law should have its way in everything.

"'At least,' said he, 'you will not have me arrested at once. It would be to your advantage as well as mine if I might leave the house for five minutes.'

"'That you may get away, or perhaps that you may conceal what you have stolen,' said I. And then, realising the dreadful position in which I was placed, I implored him to remember that not only my honour but that of one who was far greater than I was at stake; and that he threatened to raise a scandal which would *convulse* the nation. He might *avert* it all if he would but tell me what he had done with the three missing stones.

"'You may as well face the matter,' said I; 'you have been caught in the act, and no confession could make your guilt

Avert - *To ward off, prevent*

Sullenly - *Gloomily, irritatingly*

Convulse - *To shake violently*

Probed – *Investigated*

Astir – *Active, Moving*

more *heinous*. If you but make such **reparation** as is in your power, by telling us where the beryls are, all shall be forgiven and forgotten.'

"'Keep your forgiveness for those who ask for it,' he answered, turning away from me with a *sneer*. I saw that he was too hardened for any words of mine to influence him. There was but one way for it. I called in the inspector and gave him into custody. A search was made at once not only of his person but of his room and of every portion of the house where he could possibly have concealed the gems; but no trace of them could be found, nor would the wretched boy open his mouth for all our persuasions and our threats. This morning he was removed to a cell, and I, after going through all the police formalities, have hurried around to you to implore you to use your skill in **unravelling** the matter. The police have openly confessed that they can at present make nothing of it. You may go to any expense which you think necessary. I have already offered a reward of 1000 pounds. My God, what shall I do! I have lost my honour, my gems, and my son in one night. Oh, what shall I do!"

He put a hand on either side of his head and rocked himself to and fro, **droning** to himself like a child whose grief has got beyond words.

Sherlock Holmes sat silent for some few minutes, with his brows knitted and his eyes fixed upon the fire.

"Do you receive much company?" he asked.

"None save my partner with his family and an occasional friend of Arthur's. Sir George Burnwell has been several times lately. No one else, I think."

"Do you go out much in society?"

"Arthur does. Mary and I stay at home. We neither of us care for it."

"That is unusual in a young girl."

"She is of a quiet nature. Besides, she is not so very young. She is four-and-twenty."

"This matter, from what you say, seems to have been a shock to her also."

"Terrible! She is even more affected than I."

"You have neither of you any doubt as to your son's guilt?"

"How can we have when I saw him with my own eyes with the coronet in his hands."

Droning - *Humming, Buzzing*
Sneer - *To smile in making of amends for wrong or injury done*
Reparation - *In a scorn*
Heinous – *Shameful*
Unravellng – *Sorting out*

"I hardly consider that a conclusive proof. Was the remainder of the coronet at all injured?"

"Yes, it was twisted."

"Do you not think, then, that he might have been trying to straighten it?"

"God bless you! You are doing what you can for him and for me. But it is too heavy a task. What was he doing there at all? If his purpose were innocent, why did he not say so?"

"Precisely. And if he were guilty, why did he not invent a lie? His silence appears to me to cut both ways. There are several singular points about the case. What did the police think of the noise which awoke you from your sleep?"

"They considered that it might be caused by Arthur's closing his bedroom door."

"A likely story! As if a man bent on felony would slam his door so as to wake a household. What did they say, then, of the disappearance of these gems?"

"They are still sounding the *planking* and probing the furniture in the hope of finding them."

"Have they thought of looking outside the house?"

"Yes, they have shown extraordinary energy. The whole garden has already been minutely examined."

"Now, my dear sir," said Holmes. "is it not obvious to you now that this matter really strikes very much deeper than either you or the police were at first inclined to think? It appeared to you to be a simple case; to me it seems exceedingly complex. Consider what is involved by your theory. You suppose that your son came down from his bed, went, at great risk, to your dressing-room, opened your bureau, took out your coronet, broke off by main force a small portion of it, went off to some other place, concealed three gems out of the thirty-nine, with such skill that nobody can find them, and then returned with the other thirty-six into the room in which he exposed himself to the greatest danger of being discovered. I ask you now, is such a theory *tenable*?"

"But what other is there?" cried the banker with a gesture of despair. "If his motives were innocent, why does he not explain them?"

"It is our task to find that out," replied Holmes; "so now, if you please, Mr. Holder, we will set off for Streatham together, and devote an hour to glancing a little more closely into details."

Planking – *Wooden planks used to make floors*
Tenable – *Reasonable*

My friend insisted upon my accompanying them in their expedition, which I was eager enough to do, for my curiosity and sympathy were deeply stirred by the story to which we had listened. I confess that the guilt of the banker's son appeared to me to be as obvious as it did to his unhappy father, but still I had such faith in Holmes's judgement that I felt that there must be some grounds for hope as long as he was dissatisfied with the accepted explanation. He hardly spoke a word the whole way out to the southern *suburb*, but sat with his chin upon his breast and his hat drawn over his eyes, sunk in the deepest thought. Our client appeared to have taken fresh heart at the little glimpse of hope which had been presented to him, and he even broke into a ***desultory*** chat with me over his business affairs. A short railway journey and a shorter walk brought us to Fairbank, the modest residence of the great financier.

Fairbank was a good-sized square house of white stone, standing back a little from the road. A double carriage-sweep, with a snow-clad lawn, stretched down in front to two large iron gates which closed the entrance. On the right side was a small wooden thicket, which led into a narrow path between two neat hedges stretching from the road to the kitchen door, and forming the tradesmen's entrance. On the left ran a lane which led to the stables, and was not itself within the grounds at all, being a public, though little used, thoroughfare. Holmes left us standing at the door and walked slowly all around the house, across the front, down the tradesmen's path, and so around by the garden behind into the stable lane. So long was he that Mr. Holder and I went into the dining room and waited by the fire until he should return. We were sitting there in silence when the door opened and a young lady came in. She was rather above the middle height, slim, with dark hair and eyes, which seemed the darker against the absolute *pallor* of her skin. I do not think that I have ever seen such deadly paleness in a woman's face. Her lips, too, were bloodless, but her eyes were flushed with crying. As she swept silently into the room, she impressed me with a greater sense of grief than the banker had done in the morning, and it was the more striking in her as she was evidently a woman of strong character, with immense capacity for self-restraint. Disregarding my presence, she went straight to her uncle and passed her hand over his head with a sweet womanly caress.

Suburb - *An area/ district lying outside a city/town*
Desultory – *Aimless*
Pallor – *Paleness*

"You have given orders that Arthur should be liberated, have you not, dad?" she asked. "No, no, my girl, the matter must be probed to the bottom."

"But I am so sure that he is innocent. You know what woman's instincts are. I know that he has done no harm and that you will be sorry for having acted so harshly."

"Why is he silent, then, if he is innocent?"

"Who knows? Perhaps, because he was so angry that you should suspect him."

"How could I help suspecting him, when I actually saw him with the coronet in his hand?"

"Oh, but he had only picked it up to look at it. Oh, do, do take my word for it that he is innocent. Let the matter drop and say no more. It is so *dreadful* to think of our dear Arthur in prison!"

"I shall never let it drop until the gems are found – never, Mary! Your affection for Arthur blinds you as to the *awful* consequences to me. Far from hushing the thing up, I have brought a gentleman down from London to inquire more deeply into it."

"This gentleman?" she asked, facing around to me.

"No, his friend. He wished us to leave him alone. He is around in the stable lane now."

"The stable lane?" She raised her dark eyebrows. "What can he hope to find there? Ah! this, I suppose, is he. I trust, sir, that you will succeed in proving, what I feel sure is the truth, that my cousin Arthur is innocent of this crime."

"I fully share your opinion, and I trust, with you, that we may prove it," returned Holmes, going back to the mat to knock the snow from his shoes. "I believe I have the honour of addressing Miss Mary Holder. Might I ask you a question or two?"

"Pray do, sir, if it may help to clear this horrible affair up."

"You heard nothing yourself last night?"

"Nothing, until my uncle here began to speak loudly. I heard that, and I came down."

"You shut up the windows and doors the night before. Did you fasten all the windows?"

"Yes."

"Were they all fastened this morning?"

Dreadful – *Terrible*
Awful – *Unpleasant*

"Yes."

"You have a maid who has a sweetheart? I think that you remarked to your uncle last night that she had been out to see him?"

"Yes, and she was the girl who waited in the drawing room, and who may have heard uncle's remarks about the coronet."

"I see. You infer that she may have gone out to tell her sweetheart, and that the two may have planned the robbery."

"But what is the good of all these *vague* theories," cried the banker impatiently, "when I have told you that I saw Arthur with the coronet in his hands?"

"Wait a little, Mr. Holder. We must come back to that. About this girl, Miss Holder. You saw her return by the kitchen door, I presume?"

"Yes; when I went to see if the door was fastened for the night, I met her slipping in. I saw the man, too, in the gloom."

"Do you know him?"

"Oh, yes! he is the *greengrocer* who brings our vegetables round. His name is Francis Prosper."

"He stood," said Holmes, "to the left of the door – that is to say, farther up the path than is necessary to reach the door?"

"Yes, he did."

"And he is a man with a wooden leg?"

Something like fear sprang up in the young lady's expressive black eyes. "Why, you are like a magician," said she. "How do you know that?" She smiled, but there was no answering smile in Holmes's thin, eager face.

"I should be very glad now to go upstairs," said he. "I shall probably wish to go over the outside of the house again. Perhaps, I had better take a look at the lower windows before I go up."

He walked swiftly around from one to the other, pausing only at the large one which looked from the hall onto the stable lane. This he opened and made a very careful examination of the *sill* with his powerful magnifying lens. "Now we shall go upstairs," said he at last.

The banker's dressing-room was a plainly furnished little chamber, with a grey carpet, a large bureau, and a long mirror. Holmes went to the bureau first and looked hard at the lock. "Which key was used to open it?" he asked.

Sill - *A horizontal timber, block serving as a foundation of a wall*
Vague – *Unclear*
Greengrocer – *One who sells vegetables*

"That which my son himself indicated – that of the cupboard of the lumber-room."

"Have you it here?"

"That is it on the dressing-table."

Sherlock Holmes took it up and opened the bureau.

"It is a noiseless lock," said he. "It is no wonder that it did not wake you. This case, I presume, contains the coronet. We must have a look at it." He opened the case, and taking out the *diadem*, he laid it upon the table. It was a magnificent specimen of the jeweller's art, and the thirty-six stones were the finest that I have ever seen. At one side of the coronet was a cracked edge, where a corner holding three gems had been torn away.

"Now, Mr. Holder," said Holmes, "here is the corner which corresponds to that which has been so unfortunately lost. Might I beg that you will break it off."

The banker *recoiled* in horror. "I should not dream of trying," said he.

"Then I will." Holmes suddenly bent his strength upon it, but without result. "I feel it give a little," said he; "but, though I am exceptionally strong in the fingers, it would take me all my time to break it. An ordinary man could not do it. Now, what do you think would happen if I did break it, Mr. Holder? There would be a noise like a pistol shot. Do you tell me that all this happened within a few yards of your bed and that you heard nothing of it?"

"I do not know what to think. It is all dark to me."

"But perhaps it may grow lighter as we go. What do you think, Miss Holder?"

"I confess that I still share my uncle's perplexity."

"Your son had no shoes or slippers on when you saw him?"

"He had nothing on save only his trousers and shirt."

"Thank you. We have certainly been favoured with extraordinary luck during this inquiry, and it will be entirely our own fault if we do not succeed in clearing the matter up. With your permission, Mr. Holder, I shall now continue my investigations outside."

He went alone, at his own request, for he explained that any unnecessary footmarks might make his task more difficult. For an hour or more, he was at work, returning at last with his feet heavy with snow and his features as *inscrutable* as ever.

Diadem – *Crown*
Recoiled – *Moved back in horror*

"I think that I have seen now all that there is to see, Mr. Holder," said he; "I can serve you best by returning to my rooms."

"But the gems, Mr. Holmes. Where are they?"

"I cannot tell."

The banker *wrung* his hands. "I shall never see them again!" he cried. "And my son? You give me hopes?"

"My opinion is in no way altered."

"Then, for God's sake, what was this dark business which was acted in my house last night?"

"If you can call upon me at my Baker Street rooms tomorrow morning between nine and ten, I shall be happy to do what I can to make it clearer. I understand that you give me *carte blanche* to act for you, provided only that I get back the gems, and that you place no limit on the sum I may draw."

"I would give my fortune to have them back."

"Very good. I shall look into the matter between this and then. Goodbye; it is just possible that I may have to come over here again before evening."

It was obvious to me that my companion's mind was now made up about the case, although what his conclusions were was more than I could even dimly imagine. Several times during our homeward journey, I endeavoured to sound him upon the point, but he always glided away to some other topic, until at last I gave it over in despair. It was not yet three, when we found ourselves in our rooms once more. He hurried to his chamber and was down again in a few minutes dressed as a common loafer. With his collar turned up, his shiny, seedy coat, his red cravat, and his worn boots, he was a perfect sample of the class.

"I think that this should do," said he, glancing into the glass above the fireplace. "I only wish that you could come with me, Watson, but I fear that it won't do. I may be on the trail in this matter, or I may be following a *will-o'-the-wisp*, but I shall soon know which it is. I hope that I may be back in a few hours." He cut a slice of beef from the joint upon the sideboard, sandwiched it between two rounds of bread, and thrusting this rude meal into his pocket, he started off upon his expedition.

Will-o-the-wisp -
Anything that deludes,
Misleads
Wrung - *twisted*
forcibly
Inscrutable
– Unreadable,
Incomprehensible
Carte blanche *– Full*
authority

I had just finished my tea when he returned, evidently in excellent spirits, swinging an old elastic-sided boot in his hand. He *chucked* it down into a corner and helped himself to a cup of tea.

"I only looked in as I passed," said he. "I am going right on."

"Where to?"

"Oh, to the other side of the West End. It may be some time before I get back. Don't wait up for me in case I should be late."

"How are you getting on?"

"Oh, so so. Nothing to complain of. I have been out to Streatham since I saw you last, but I did not call at the house. It is a very sweet little problem, and I would not have missed it for a good deal. However, I must not sit gossiping here, but must get these disreputable clothes off and return to my highly respectable self."

I could see by his manner that he had stronger reasons for satisfaction than his words alone would imply. His eyes twinkled, and there was even a touch of colour upon his *sallow* cheeks. He hastened upstairs, and a few minutes later I, heard the slam of the hall door, which told me that he was off once more upon his *congenial* hunt.

I waited until midnight, but there was no sign of his return, so I retired to my room. It was no uncommon thing for him to be away for days and nights on end when he was hot upon a scent, so that his lateness caused me no surprise. I do not know at what hour he came in, but when I came down to breakfast in the morning, there he was with a cup of coffee in one hand and the paper in the other, as fresh and trim as possible.

"You will excuse my beginning without you, Watson," said he, "but you remember that our client has rather an early appointment this morning."

"Why, it is after nine now," I answered. "I should not be surprised if that were he. I thought I heard a ring."

It was, indeed, our friend, the financier. I was shocked by the change which had come over him, for his face which was naturally of a broad and massive mould, was now pinched and fallen in, while his hair seemed to me at least a shade whiter. He entered with a *weariness* and *lethargy* which was even more painful than his violence of the morning before,

Chucked - *To toss*
Sallow – *Sickly*
Congenial – *Friendly*

and he dropped heavily into the armchair which I pushed forward for him.

"I do not know what I have done to be so severely tried," said he. "Only two days ago, I was a happy and prosperous man, without a care in the world. Now I am left to a lonely and dishonoured age. One sorrow comes *close upon the heels* of another. My niece, Mary, has deserted me."

"Deserted you?"

"Yes. Her bed this morning had not been slept in, her room was empty, and a note for me lay upon the hall table. I had said to her last night, in sorrow and not in anger, that if she had married my boy, all might have been well with him. Perhaps, it was *thoughtless* of me to say so. It is to that remark that she refers in this note:

"'MY DEAREST UNCLE,

"'I feel that I have brought trouble upon you, and that if I had acted differently, this terrible misfortune might never have occurred. I cannot, with this thought in my mind, ever again be happy under your roof, and I feel that I must leave you forever. Do not worry about my future, for that is provided for; and, above all, do not search for me, for it will be fruitless labour and an ill-service to me.

"'In life or in death, I am ever your loving

"'MARY.'

"What could she mean by that note, Mr. Holmes? Do you think it points to suicide?"

"No, no, nothing of the kind. It is perhaps the best possible solution. I trust, Mr. Holder, that you are nearing the end of your troubles."

"Ha! You say so! You have heard something, Mr. Holmes; you have learned something! Where are the gems?"

"You would not think 1000 pounds apiece an excessive sum for them?"

"I would pay ten."

Close upon the heels – *Following somebody*
Thoughtless – *Unkind*

"That would be unnecessary. Three thousand will cover the matter. And there is a little reward, I fancy. Have you your check-book? Here is a pen. Better make it out for 4000 pounds."

With a dazed face the banker made out the required check. Holmes walked over to his desk, took out a little triangular piece of gold with three gems in it, and threw it down upon the table.

With a shriek of joy our client clutched it up.

"You have it!" he *gasped*. "I am saved! I am saved!"

The reaction of joy was as passionate as his grief had been, and he hugged his recovered gems to his bosom.

"There is one other thing you owe, Mr. Holder," said Sherlock Holmes rather sternly.

"Owe!" He caught up a pen. "Name the sum, and I will pay it."

"No, the debt is not to me. You owe a very humble apology to that noble lad, your son, who has carried himself in this matter as I should be proud to see my own son do, should I ever chance to have one."

"Then it was not Arthur who took them?"

"I told you yesterday, and I repeat today, that it was not."

"You are sure of it! Then let us hurry to him at once to let him know that the truth is known."

"He knows it already. When I had cleared it all up, I had an interview with him, and finding that he would not tell me the story, I told it to him, on which he had to confess that I was right and to add the very few details which were not yet quite clear to me. Your news of this morning, however, may open his lips."

"For heaven's sake, tell me, then, what is this extraordinary mystery!"

"I will do so, and I will show you the steps by which I reached it. And let me say to you, first, that which it is hardest for me to say and for you to hear: there has been an understanding between Sir George Burnwell and your niece, Mary. They have now fled together."

"My Mary? Impossible!"

"It is unfortunately more than possible; it is certain. Neither you nor your son knew the true character of this man when you admitted him into your family circle. He is one of the most dangerous men in England – a ruined gambler, an absolutely desperate villain, a man without heart or *conscience*. Your niece knew nothing of such men. When

Gasped – *Panted*
Conscience – *Sense of right and wrong*

he breathed his vows to her, as he had done to a hundred before her, she flattered herself that she alone had touched his heart. The devil knows best what he said, but at least, she became his tool and was in the habit of seeing him nearly every evening."

"I cannot, and I will not, believe it!" cried the banker with an *ashen* face.

"I will tell you, then, what occurred in your house last night. Your niece, when you had, as she thought, gone to your room, slipped down and talked to her lover through the window which leads into the stable lane. His footmarks had pressed right through the snow, so long had he stood there. She told him of the coronet. His wicked lust for gold *kindled* at the news, and he bent her to his will. I have no doubt that she loved you, but there are women in whom the love of a lover extinguishes all other loves, and I think that she must have been one. She had hardly listened to his instructions when she saw you coming downstairs, on which she closed the window rapidly and told you about one of the servants' escapade with her wooden-legged lover, which was all perfectly true.

"Your boy, Arthur, went to bed after his interview with you but he slept badly on account of his uneasiness about his club debts. In the middle of the night, he heard a soft *tread* pass his door, so he rose and, looking out, was surprised to see his cousin walking very stealthily along the passage until she disappeared into your dressing-room. *Petrified* with astonishment, the lad slipped on some clothes and waited there in the dark to see what would come of this strange affair. Presently, she emerged from the room again, and in the light of the passage-lamp, your son saw that she carried the precious coronet in her hands. She passed down the stairs, and he, thrilling with horror, ran along and slipped behind the curtain near your door, whence he could see what passed in the hall beneath. He saw her stealthily open the window, hand out the coronet to someone in the gloom, and then closing it once more, hurry back to her room, passing quite close to where he stood hid behind the curtain.

"As long as she was on the scene, he could not take any action without a horrible exposure of the woman whom he loved. But the instant that she was gone, he realised how crushing a misfortune this would be for you, and how all-important it was to set it right. He rushed down, just as he

Extinguishes - *To put out a fire*
Petrified - *Benumbed or paralysed*
Ashen – *Pale*
Kindled – *Started burning*

Greatest Adventure Stories of Sherlock Holmes - 2

was, in his bare feet, opened the window, sprang out into the snow, and ran down the lane, where he could see a dark figure in the moonlight. Sir George Burnwell tried to get away, but Arthur caught him, and there was a struggle between them, your lad *tugging* at one side of the coronet, and his opponent at the other. In the *scuffle*, your son struck Sir George and cut him over the eye. Then something suddenly snapped, and your son, finding that he had the coronet in his hands, rushed back, closed the window, *ascended* to your room, and had just observed that the coronet had been twisted in the struggle and was endeavouring to straighten it when you appeared upon the scene."

"Is it possible?" gasped the banker.

"You then roused his anger by calling him names at a moment when he felt that he had deserved your warmest thanks. He could not explain the true state of affairs without betraying one who certainly deserved little enough consideration at his hands. He took the more *chivalrous* view, however, and preserved her secret."

"And that was why she shrieked and fainted when she saw the coronet," cried Mr. Holder. "Oh, my God! what a blind fool I have been! And his asking to be allowed to go out for five minutes! The dear fellow wanted to see if the missing piece were at the scene of the struggle. How cruelly I have misjudged him!'

"When I arrived at the house," continued Holmes, "I at once went very carefully around it to observe if there were any traces in the snow which might help me. I knew that none had fallen since the evening before, and also that there had been a strong frost to preserve impressions. I passed along the tradesmen's path, but found it all trampled down and indistinguishable. Just beyond it, however, at the far side of the kitchen door, a woman had stood and talked with a man, whose round impressions on one side showed that he had a wooden leg. I could even tell that they had been disturbed, for the woman had run back swiftly to the door, as was shown by the deep toe and light heel marks, while Wooden-leg had waited a little, and then had gone away. I thought at the time that this might be the maid and her sweetheart, of whom you had already spoken to me, and inquiry showed it was so. I passed around the garden without seeing anything more than random tracks, which I took to be the police; but when I got

Scuffle – Quarrel
Ascended – Rose up, Climp

into the stable lane, a very long and complex story was written in the snow in front of me.

"There was a double line of tracks of a booted man, and a second double line which I saw with delight belonged to a man with naked feet. I was at once convinced from what you had told me that the latter was your son. The first had walked both ways, but the other had run swiftly, and as his tread was marked in places over the *depression* of the boot, it was obvious that he had passed after the other. I followed them up and found, they led to the hall window, where the Boots had worn all the snow away while waiting. Then I walked to the other end, which was a hundred yards or more down the lane. I saw where the Boots had faced around, where the snow was cut up as though there had been a struggle, and, finally, where a few drops of blood had fallen, to show me that I was not mistaken. Boots had then run down the lane, and another little *smudge* of blood showed that it was he who had been hurt. When he came to the highroad at the other end, I found that the pavement had been cleared, so there was an end to that clue.

"On entering the house, however, I examined, as you remember, the sill and framework of the hall window with my lens, and I could at once see that someone had passed out. I could distinguish the outline of an *instep* where the wet foot had been placed in coming in. I was then beginning to be able to form an opinion as to what had occurred. A man had waited outside the window; someone had brought the gems; the deed had been overseen by your son; he had pursued the thief; had struggled with him; they had each tugged at the coronet, their united strength causing injuries which neither alone could have effected. He had returned with the prize, but had left a fragment in the grasp of his opponent. So far I was clear. The question now was, who was the man and who was it brought him the coronet?

"It is an old maxim of mine that when you have excluded the impossible, whatever remains, however *improbable*, must be the truth. Now, I knew that it was not you who had brought it down, so there only remained your niece and the maids. But if it were the maids, why should your son allow himself to be accused in their place? There could be no possible reason. As he loved his cousin, however, there was an excellent explanation why he should retain her secret – the more so as the secret

Improbable -
Unlikely to be true
Smudge - *A dirty mark or smear*
Depression – *Misery*
Instep – *The top part of the foot between the ankle and toes*

was a disgraceful one. When I remembered that you had seen her at that window, and how she had fainted on seeing the coronet again, my conjecture became a certainty.

"And who could it be who was her *confederate*? A lover evidently, for who else could outweigh the love and gratitude which she must feel to you? I knew that you went out little, and that your circle of friends was a very limited one. But among them was Sir George Burnwell. I had heard of him before as being a man of evil reputation among women. It must have been he who wore those boots and retained the missing gems. Even though he knew that Arthur had discovered him, he might still *flatter* himself that he was safe, for the lad could not say a word without compromising his own family.

"Well, your own good sense will suggest what measures I took next. I went in the shape of a loafer to Sir George's house, managed to pick up an acquaintance with his *valet*, learned that his master had cut his head the night before, and, finally, at the expense of six shillings, made all sure by buying a pair of his cast-off shoes. With these I journeyed down to Streatham and saw that they exactly fitted the tracks."

"I saw an ill-dressed *vagabond* in the lane yesterday evening," said Mr. Holder.

"Precisely. It was I. I found that I had my man, so I came home and changed my clothes. It was a delicate part which I had to play then, for I saw that a *prosecution* must be avoided to avert *scandal*, and I knew that so *astute* a villain would see that our hands were tied in the matter. I went and saw him. At first, of course, he denied everything. But when I gave him every particular that had occurred, he tried to *bluster* and took down a life-preserver from the wall. I knew my man, however, and I clapped a pistol to his head before he could strike. Then he became a little more reasonable. I told him that we would give him a price for the stones he held, 1000 pounds apiece. That brought out the first signs of grief that he had shown. 'Why, dash it all!' said he, 'I've let them go at six hundred for the three!' I soon managed to get the address of the receiver who had them, on promising him that there would be no prosecution. Off I set to him, and after much *chaffering*, I got our stones at 1000 pounds apiece. Then I looked in upon your son, told him that all was right, and eventually, got to my bed about two o'clock, after what I may call a really hard day's work."

Astute - *Keen and clever*

Scandal - *A disgraceful action*

Prosecution - *Law or law making body*

Vagabond - *Nomadic*

Valet - *A male servant*

Bluster – *Threaten*

Chaffering – *Haggling*

"A day which has saved England from a great public scandal," said the banker, rising. "Sir, I cannot find words to thank you, but you shall not find me *ungrateful* for what you have done. Your skill has indeed exceeded all that I have heard of it. And now I must fly to my dear boy to *apologize* to him for the wrong which I have done him. As to what you tell me of poor Mary, it goes to my very heart. Not even your skill can inform me where she is now."

"I think that we may safely say," returned Holmes, "that she is wherever Sir George Burnwell is. It is equally certain, too, that whatever her *sins* are, they will soon receive a more than sufficient punishment."

Apologise - *To beg for forgiveness*
Sins - *Bad deeds*
Ungrateful - *Unappreciative, Thankless*

Food For Thought

What would have happened if Holmes would not have noticed the double line of tracks of a booted man, and a scond double line of a man with naked feet in the stable lane of Mr. Holder's house? Would it been possible for Holmes to catch the real culprit then? What woud have been the fate of Arthur?

An Understanding

Q. 1. Why did the author, Sir Arthur Conan Doyle feel that Mr. Alexander Holder was a mad man at first when he saw Mr. Holder from his bow-window?

Ans. _____

_____

_____

_____

_____

Q. 2. Why wa Mr. Holder behaving in such an natural manner? What was wrong with him?

Ans. _____

_____

_____

_____

_____

Q. 3. Describe the appearance and character sketch of Mary, the niece of Mr. Holder. How did it contrast with the character of Arthur, Mr. Holder's son?

Ans. _____

_____

_____

_____

_____

Q. 4. "Your son had no shoes or slippers on when you saw him?" Why did Holmes ask the above question to Mr. Holder? Why was the question so important in solving this case?

Ans. _____

_____

_____

_____

_____

SELF-IMPROVEMENT/PERSONALITY DEVELOPMENT

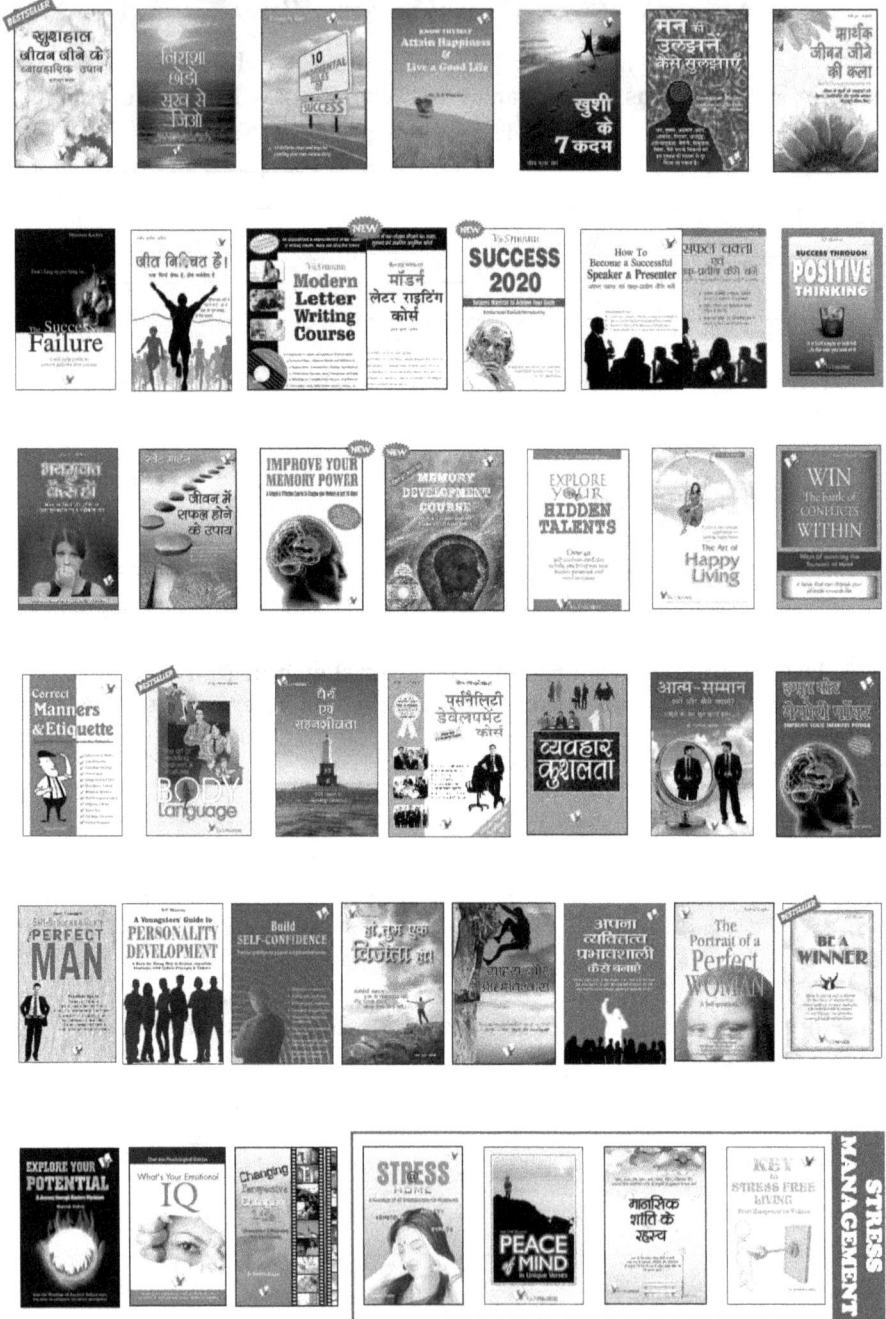

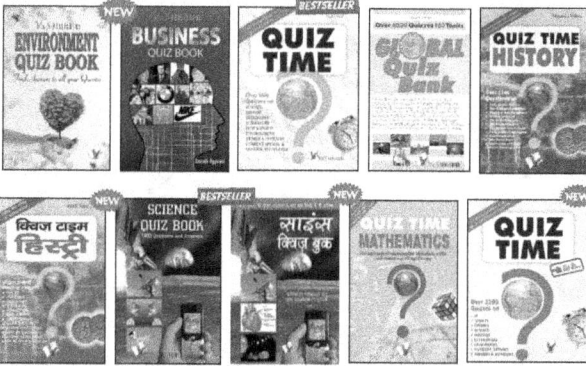

QUIZ BOOKS

ENGLISH IMPROVEMENT

OTHERS LANGUAGE

ACTIVITIES BOOK

QUOTES/SAYINGS

BIOGRAPHIES/CHILDREN SCIENCE LIBRARY

COMPUTER BOOKS

All books available at www.vspublishers.com

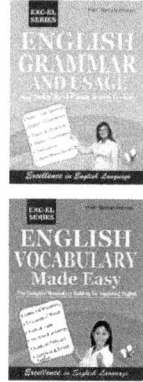

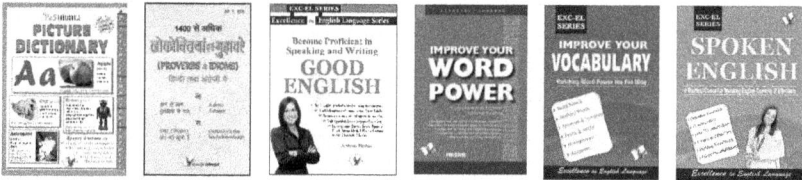

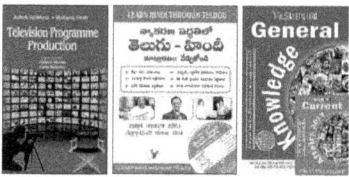

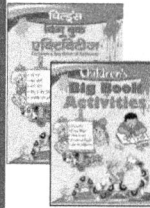

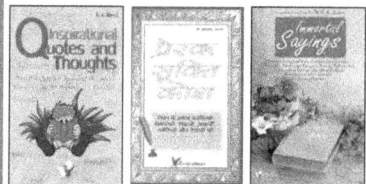

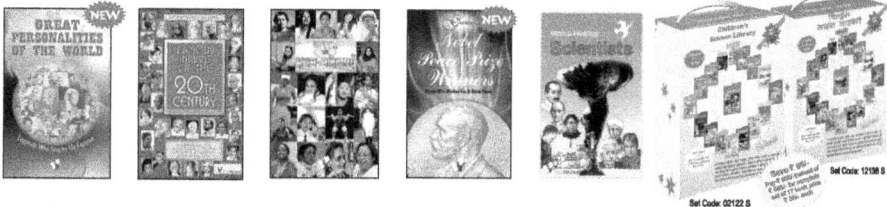

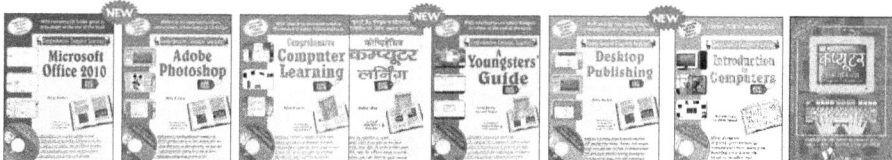

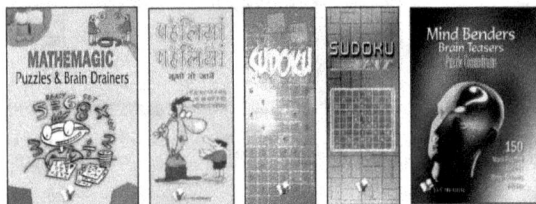

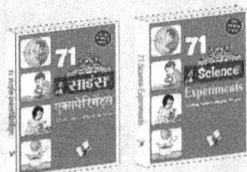

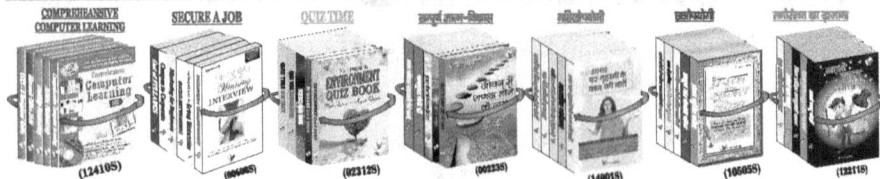

STUDENT DEVELOPMENT/LEARNING

POPULAR SCIENCE

PUZZLES

DRAWING BOOKS

VALUE PACKS

(124105)   (00460S)   (023125)   (00233S)   (140015)   (105055)   (132115)

All books available at www.vspublishers.com

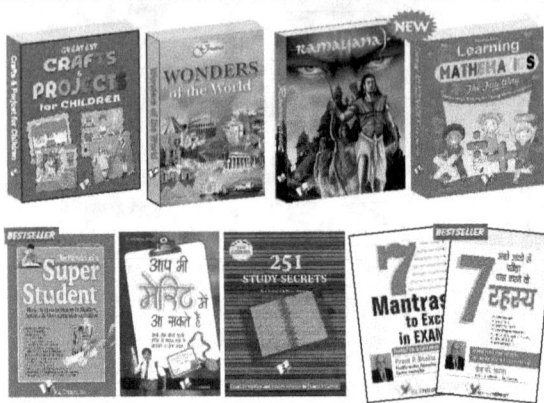

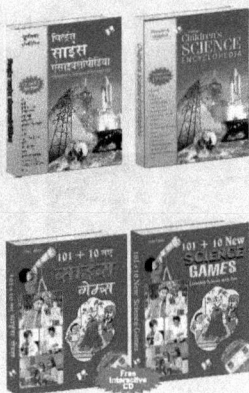

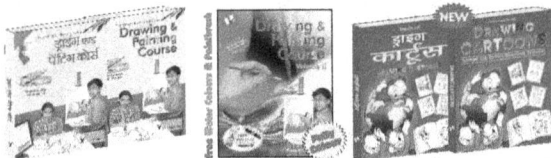

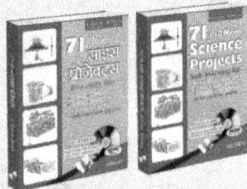

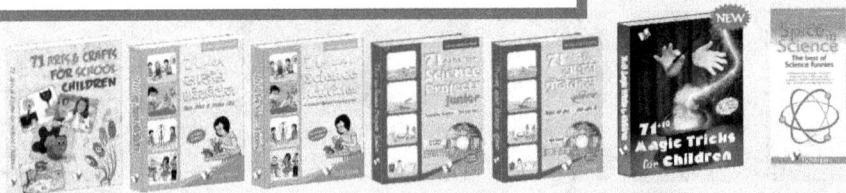

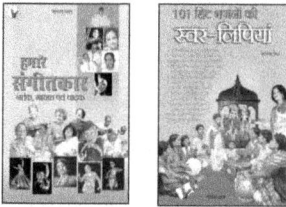

HINDI LITERATURE

MUSIC (संगीत)

MAGIC & FACT (जादू एवं तथ्य)

ACADEMIC BOOKS

TALES & STORIES

All Books Fully Coloured

MYSTERIES (रहस्य)

All books available at **www.vspublishers.com**

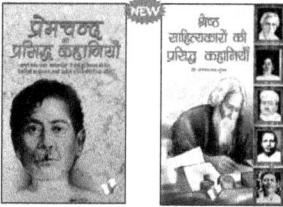

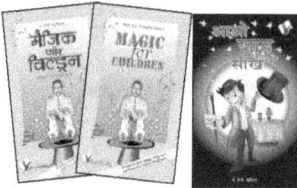

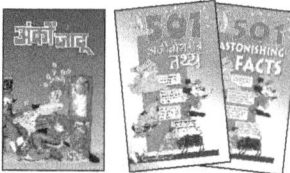

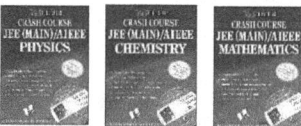

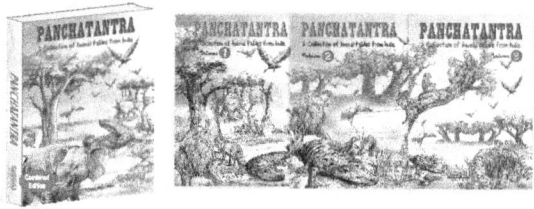

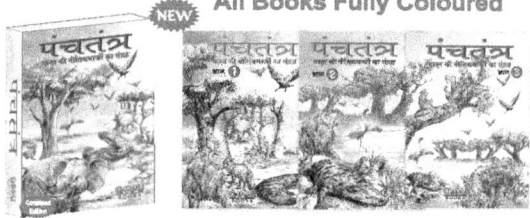

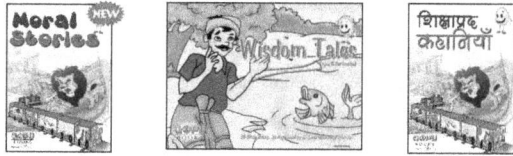

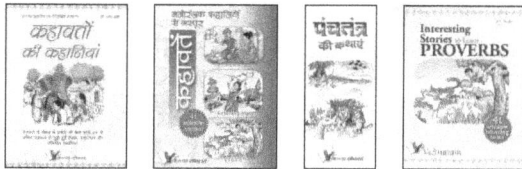

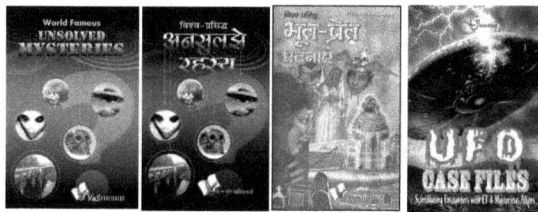

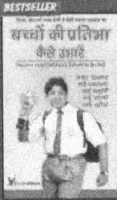

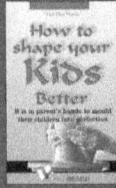

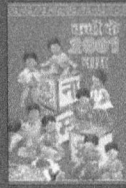

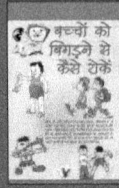

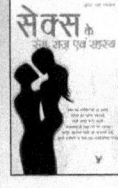

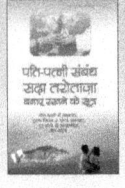

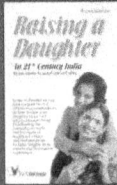

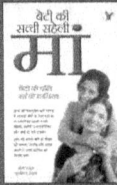

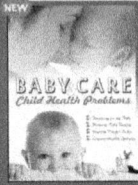

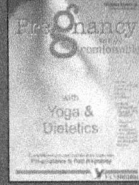

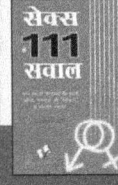

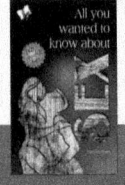

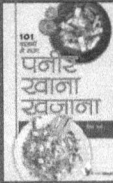

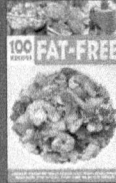

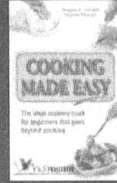

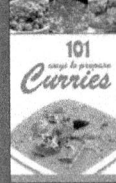

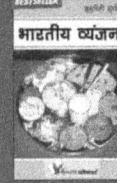

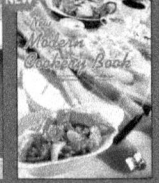

PARENTING

FAMILY & RELATIONS

COOKING

HOUSEKEEPING

WOMEN ORIENTED

All books available at www.vspublishers.com

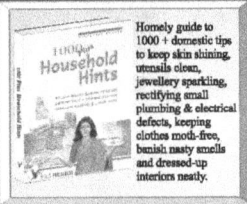

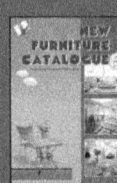

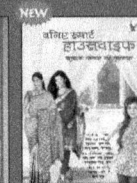

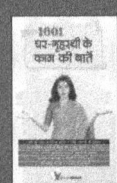

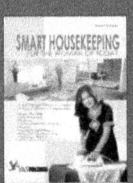

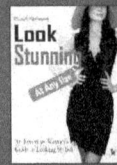

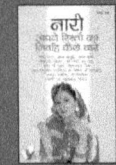

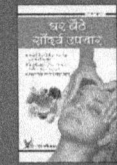

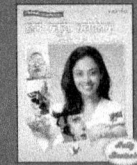

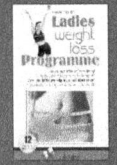

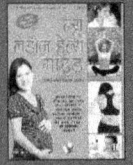

GENERAL HEALTH & BEAUTY CARE

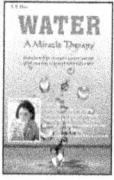

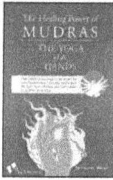

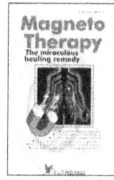

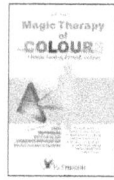

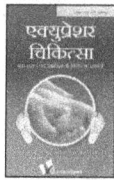

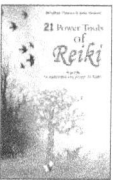

ALTERNATIV THERAPY

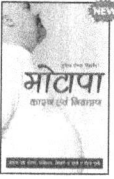

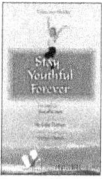

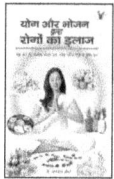

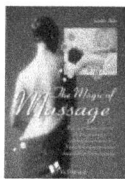

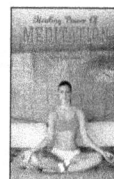

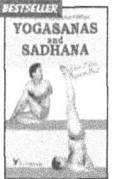

WATER — A Miracle Therapy
The Healing Power of MUDRAS — THE YOGA of GANDS
Magneto Therapy — The miraculous healing remedy
Magic Therapy of COLOUR
एक्यूप्रेशर चिकित्सा
21 Power Tools of Reiki

FITNESS

मोटापा
Stay Youthful Forever
योग और भोजन से रोगों का इलाज
The Magic of Massage
Healing Power of MEDITATION
YOGASANAS and SADHANA — BESTSELLER

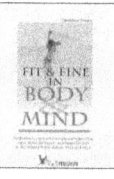

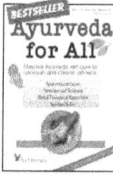

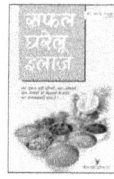

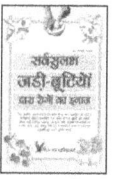

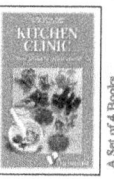

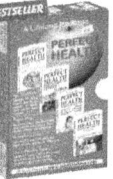

PERFECT HEALTH & AYURVEDA

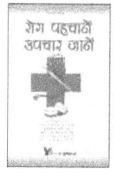

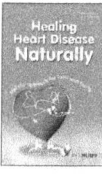

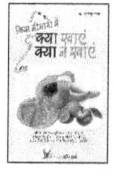

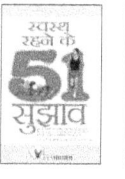

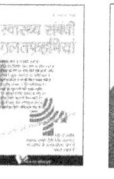

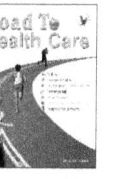

FIT & FINE IN BODY MIND
Ayurveda for All — BESTSELLER
सफल घरेलू इलाज
सर्वसुलभ जड़ी-बूटियाँ द्वारा रोगों का इलाज
KITCHEN CLINIC
PERFECT HEALTH — BESTSELLER — A Set of 4 Books

DISEASES & COMMON AILMENTS

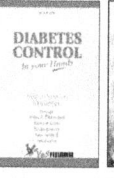

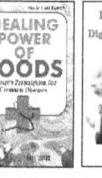

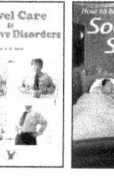

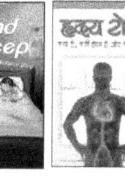

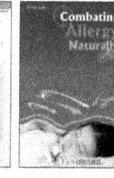

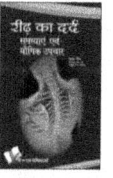

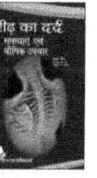

रोग पहचानो उपचार जानो
Healing Heart Disease Naturally
दिल की बीमारी में क्या खाएं क्या न खाएं
स्वस्थ रहने के 51 सुझाव
स्वास्थ्य संबंधी गलतफहमियां
Road To Health Care

DIABETES CONTROL In your Hands
HEALING POWER OF FOODS — Nature's Prescription for Common Illnesses
Bowel Care & Digestive Disorders
Sound Sleep
हृदय रोग
Combating Allergy Naturally
रीढ़ का दर्द — समस्याएं एवं योगिक उपचार

All books available at www.vspublishers.com

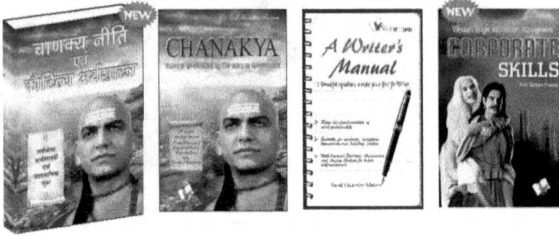

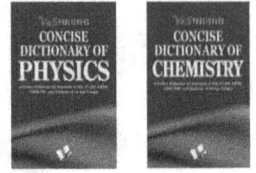

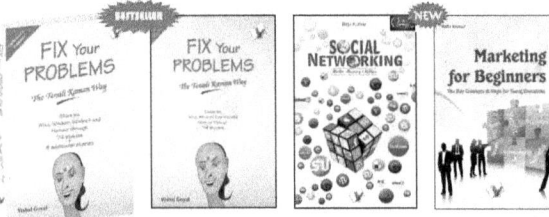

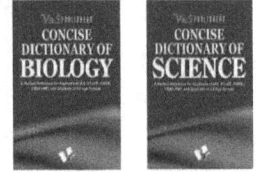

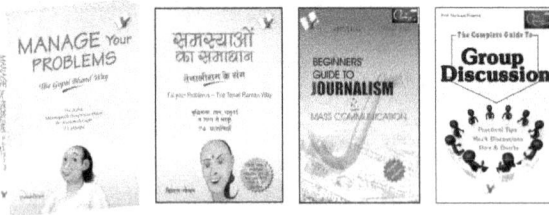

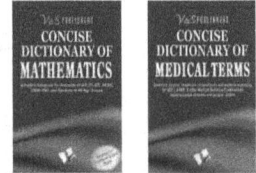

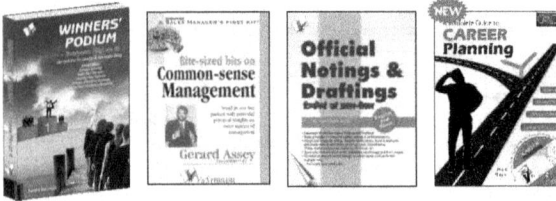

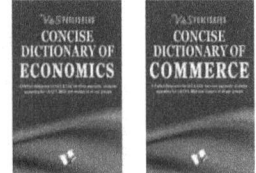

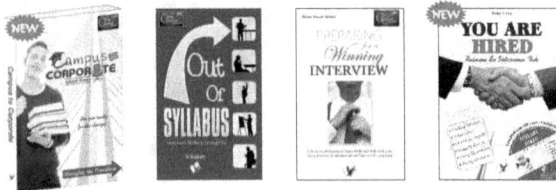

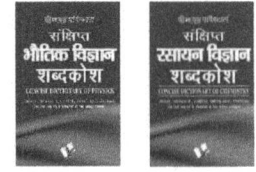

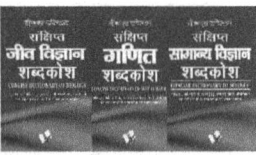

All books available at **www.vspublishers.com**

www.ingramcontent.com/pod-product-compliance
Lightning Source LLC
Chambersburg PA
CBHW050713280326
41926CB00088B/3011